A Lean Guide to Transforming Healthcare

Also available from ASQ Quality Press:

Lean-Six Sigma for Healthcare: A Senior Leader Guide to Improving Cost and Throughput
Chip Caldwell, Jim Brexler, and Tom Gillem

Improving Healthcare with Control Charts: Basic and Advanced SPC Methods and Case Studies
Raymond G. Carey

The Manager's Guide to Six Sigma in Healthcare: Practical Tips and Tools for Improvement
Robert Barry and Amy C. Smith

Stop Rising Healthcare Costs Using Toyota Lean Production Methods: 38 Steps for Improvement
Robert Chalice

The Six Sigma Book for Healthcare: Improving Outcomes by Reducing Errors
Robert Barry, Amy Murcko, and Clifford Brubaker

Lean Kaizen: A Simplified Approach to Process Improvements
George Alukal and Anthony Manos

5S for Service Organizations and Offices: A Lean Look at Improvements
Debashis Sarkar

Root Cause Analysis: Simplified Tools and Techniques, Second Edition
Bjørn Andersen and Tom Fagerhaug

The Quality Toolbox, Second Edition
Nancy R. Tague

Making Change Work: Practical Tools for Overcoming Human Resistance to Change
Brien Palmer

The Path to Profitable Measures: 10 Steps to Feedback That Fuels Performance
Mark W. Morgan

To request a complimentary catalog of ASQ Quality Press publications, call 800-248-1946, or visit our Web site at http://qualitypress.asq.org.

A Lean Guide to Transforming Healthcare

How to Implement Lean Principles in Hospitals, Medical Offices, Clinics, and Other Healthcare Organizations

THOMAS G. ZIDEL

ASQ Quality Press
Milwaukee, Wisconsin

American Society for Quality, Quality Press, Milwaukee, WI 53203
© 2006 by ASQ
All rights reserved. Published 2006.
Printed in the United States of America.

12   11   10   09   08   07   06   5   4   3   2   1

Library of Congress Cataloging-in-Publication Data

Zidel, Tom, 1949-
  A lean guide to transforming healthcare : how to implement lean principles in
  hospitals, medical offices, clinics, and other healthcare organizations / Tom Zidel.
      p.; cm.
  Includes bibliographical references and index.
  ISBN-13: 978-0-87389-701-3 (alk. paper)
  ISBN-10: 0-87389-701-3 (alk. paper)
  1. Health services administration. 2. Industrial efficiency. 3. Just-in-time systems. I. Title.
  [DNLM: 1. Delivery of Health Care--organization & administration. 2. Efficiency,
  Organizational. 3. Health Care Reform--methods. W 84.1 Z64L 2006]

  RA971.Z53 2006
  362.11068--dc22
                                2006022782

Publisher: William A. Tony
Acquisitions Editor: Matt T. Meinholz
Project Editor: Paul O'Mara
Production Administrator: Randall Benson

ASQ Mission: The American Society for Quality advances individual,
organizational, and community excellence worldwide through learning, quality
improvement, and knowledge exchange.

Attention Bookstores, Wholesalers, Schools, and Corporations: ASQ Quality Press
books, videotapes, audiotapes, and software are available at quantity discounts
with bulk purchases for business, educational, or instructional use. For information,
please contact ASQ Quality Press at 800-248-1946, or write to ASQ Quality Press,
P.O. Box 3005, Milwaukee, WI 53201-3005.

To place orders or to request a free copy of the ASQ Quality Press Publications
Catalog, including ASQ membership information, call 800-248-1946. Visit our
Web site at www.asq.org or http://qualitypress.asq.org.

∞ Printed on acid-free paper

Quality Press
600 N. Plankinton Avenue
Milwaukee, Wisconsin 53203
Call toll free 800-248-1946
Fax 414-272-1734
www.asq.org
http://qualitypress.asq.org
http://standardsgroup.asq.org
E-mail: authors@asq.org

ASQ
AMERICAN SOCIETY
FOR QUALITY™

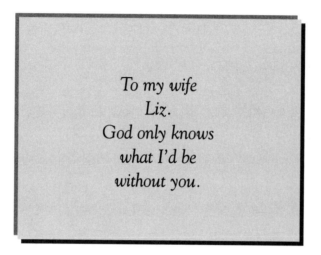

To my wife
Liz.
God only knows
what I'd be
without you.

Contents

LIST OF ILLUSTRATIONS

FIGURES

TABLES

FOREWORD

Healthcare leaders, policy makers, employers, and patients wrestle mightily with an industry that consumes a greater and greater portion of the economy while falling farther away from meeting basic (although rising) expectations regarding safety, quality, and customer service. Moreover, at the same time that evidence mounts to support the relationship between human resources and clinical quality, the industry is faced with unprecedented shortages of critical human capital such as nursing expertise.

As a consumer, practicing physician, and healthcare quality executive, I find it striking that it is still possible to see an abundance of time and effort spent waiting, working around established processes, and correcting defects in service, even in the face of these shortages. I know that I ought not be surprised, given the complexity of care across time and space, the involvement of countless individuals in caring for a typical hospital patient, and the variation and ambiguity in decision making, processes, and information flow needed to coordinate care.

Recognizing that we can and must do better, organizations are turning to a variety of improvement tools and methodologies to enhance reliability and efficiency. To a great extent, these explorations have paralleled quality initiatives in other industries: Total Quality Management, Six Sigma, and Business Process Reengineering have found followers in the healthcare sector.

Improvement efforts must address three complimentary objectives: improving reliability, enhancing efficiency, and promoting organizational acceptance. The *lean* approach to improvement proves to be an effective set of tools for achieving these three objectives. By seeking to identify waste in the processes we use to accomplish our work, including the waste attributable to failures and defects, *lean* thinking addresses both reliability and efficiency directly. Engaging employees directly in a process of data-driven experimentation and experiential learning, *lean* approaches hold the promise of greater organizational acceptance for changes in work processes.

A *lean* transformation represents a paradigm shift in the way we view work and in the approaches we use to improve. Tom Zidel's *A Lean Guide to Transforming Healthcare* provides readers a clear and detailed roadmap for this kind of transformation. It also presents a practical set of tools for seeing and seizing opportunities to do things better. As organizations seek to fuel improvement, they wrestle with the challenge of moving from one approach, such as Six Sigma, to another, such as *lean*. Rather than promoting an "either-or" approach to improvement, Tom's guide illustrates how complimentary and easily integrated a *lean* approach may be with Six Sigma.

Not knowing where to start or how to proceed can be considerable barriers to initiating improvement efforts, particularly when the objective knowingly requires a paradigm shift and new methods. *A Lean Guide to Transforming Healthcare* is just the field manual necessary for getting us moving on the path.

Michael Apkon, MBA, Ph.D, MD,

Dr. Apkon is VP of Performance Management for Yale-New Haven Health Systems, Vice Chairman of Pediatrics, Medical Director of the Pediatric Intensive Care Unit, and Medical Director of the Yale-New Haven Health System New Clinical Program Development Fund. He is an Associate Professor at both the Yale School of Medicine and the Yale School of Management. He received an M.B.A. from the Yale School of Management, and an M.D. and Ph.D. in Neural Sciences from Washington University.

PREFACE

During my tenure in healthcare I have attended many seminars on the subject of Lean in healthcare. All of these seminars focused on the benefits of Lean to the healthcare organization, but failed to answer the two most important questions the attendees had relative to Lean. First, "What exactly does it mean to be a lean organization?" Second, and more importantly, "How do we implement Lean in our organization?" Even my own attempts to convey the principles, tools, and techniques of lean to individuals requesting clarification would often lead to more confusion and more questions: "What is a kanban?" "Who implements standard work?" "Are you saying that what I do everyday is non-value-added?" "My department is fine; it's the other departments that are causing my problems." "I only have two people in my department, I'm already lean!" The need for an organized and detailed explanation of lean principles became glaringly obvious.

A Lean Guide to Transforming Healthcare is an implementation manual for lean tools and principles in a healthcare environment. The book begins with an illustrative exercise that clearly exemplifies the basic underlying principle of lean. In addition, the need for change in healthcare, a call to action, and the level of commitment required for a successful lean transformation are discussed early on.

The need for change in healthcare has never been more apparent than it is today. Healthcare is the country's largest industry. It's poised for exponential growth as baby boomers reach their sixties, yet external influences make it more and more difficult for hospitals to prosper.

Lean is a growth strategy, a survival strategy, and an improvement strategy. The goal of lean, first and foremost, is to provide value to the patient/customer and in so doing eliminate the delays, overcrowding, and frustration associated with the existing care delivery system. Lean creates a better working environment where what is supposed to happen does happen, on time, every time. It allows clinicians to spend more of their time caring for patients and improves the quality of care these patients receive. A lean organization values its employees and encourages their involvement in organizational initiatives. This, in turn, sustains hospital-wide quality improvements.

Manufacturing and service organizations all over the world have been successfully implementing lean principles and reaping enormous benefits. Lean principles are now being successfully implemented in hospitals with great success. The opportunities for lean in the healthcare environment are limitless.

Implementation requires a new way of looking at the care delivery process, a paradigm shift that will transform the way value is delivered to the patient/customer. To achieve a lean transformation, a thorough understanding of lean principles, as well as knowledge of lean tools and their application in a healthcare environment, is essential. This book provides all of these elements and is meant to be used as an implementation guide.

Chapter 3 provides a road map for lean implementation, from strategic planning to creating flow. The heart of the book is dedicated to the tools of lean, beginning with Value Stream Mapping and 5S, which comprise one of the key concepts of a lean transformation: user-friendliness. The book progresses with explanations of the most common techniques used for lean implementation, including an introduction to Six Sigma. It culminates with a chapter explaining how these tools all come together in a lean event. The final chapter is a call to action.

This is not a book to be read and forgotten, nor is it meant to sit on a bookshelf as another addition to an impressive but underutilized collection of how-to books. As the name implies, it is a guide, a companion to be referenced again and again as the organization moves forward with its lean transformation. If I were to visit an organization, I would hope to see this book torn and tattered from excessive use, dog-eared, bookmarked, annotated with notes in the margins and sections vigorously highlighted.

There are always inherent risks associated with trying something new, but as the saying goes, "the longest journey begins with a single step." Take that first step toward becoming a lean organization.

ACKNOWLEDGEMENTS

Many thanks go to all the amazing people who not only showed patience with my apparent lack of knowledge and difficulty in grasping the concepts associated with the healthcare environment, but who also supported and encouraged my endeavors. I have never worked with a group of people as caring and selfless as the people I have met in healthcare.

Many thanks go to the group from SCARI-QA, Sue Simons, Diane Miller, Robin Green, and Evelyn Carusillo.

I also wish to thank MaryBeth Bednarz, Linda Mulvihill, Kathleen Woods, and Bill Taft for their continued friendship and trust.

Thanks to Jim Cutler and Mark Hamel of Moffitt Associates for affording me the opportunity to continue my pursuit of lean implementation in healthcare.

Thank you to the Yale-New Haven Health System for allowing me to come into their organization and demonstrate the value of lean. Especially, thank you to Michael Apkon, MBA, M.D., Ph.D. and Michael Pepe, Ph. D. who together spearheaded the initiative to bring lean to Yale-New Haven Health Systems.

Finally, I would like to thank my parents who have always supported, loved, and provided for my brother and me.

Some photos and text used in this book also appeared in the *Journal of Healthcare Quality*, Web Exclusive, Vol.28, No 1, pp W1-7-W1-15.

INTRODUCTION

On Monday, May 1, 2000, I sat in the conference hall of a hospital where I had accepted a newly created position as Director of Continuous Improvement. The same thought kept running through my head: "What was I thinking?" The closest thing I had to what could be considered hospital experience was my tour of duty as a medic during the Vietnam War, which was thirty years prior. I kept telling myself that a hospital was no different from any other organization and everything would be fine. Was I wrong! Healthcare is most definitely in a class all its own.

To complicate my arrival, I began my new position in the wake of destruction left by consultants who, under the guise of lean, issued a staff reduction that left almost everyone in the hospital bitter and resistant to change, especially change generated by lean implementation. Once again, the thought ran through my head, "What was I thinking?"

I immediately recognized that my first task was to overcome this resistance to change, which I knew would require much effort on my part. I expect that few hospitals will experience this heightened level of resistance, although most organizations will undoubtedly experience some. Therefore, I felt it appropriate to preface this book with an analogy regarding resistance to change.

Like the earth, the existing care delivery system has a gravitational pull. Whenever we try to do things differently, there is a pull at us to cling to the familiar and embrace those methods with which we feel comfortable. Eventually this pull gravitates us right back to our old way of doing things and we return to the status quo. Just as it takes tremendous force to break away from the gravitational pull of the earth, it takes great determination to break away from the status quo.

The space shuttle uses three main engines fueled by a huge external fuel tank combined with two solid rocket boosters to generate more than seven and a half million pounds of thrust in an effort to break through the earth's gravitational pull. A news anchor once declared during an early launch, "We're not sure if the rocket is going to go up or if Florida is going to go down." This initial force can be likened to the commitment and tenacity required on the part of senior administration and management in launching a lean initiative.

After approximately two minutes the fuel in the two solid rocket boosters is exhausted and the boosters are jettisoned. This is interesting because at this point the space shuttle has reached the edge of the earth's atmosphere. It is still within the gravitational pull of the earth, but because the air is thin or non-existent there is no friction to slow the spacecraft down. The same is true with change. At some point after launch, when members of the organization begin to see improvement and to believe that this initiative won't be "just another program," resistance subsides and eventually becomes non-existent.

Again, something very interesting happens. Once the boosters have been jettisoned, the three main engines continue to burn for another six and a half minutes, consuming the fuel in the external tank and making the spacecraft lighter. This is important because the spacecraft needs to accelerate to a velocity of 25,000 miles per hour, almost twenty-three times faster than a speeding bullet. Likewise, with lean, once the resistance to change subsides, the rate at which lean tools and concepts spread throughout the organization will accelerate at a tremendous rate.

When the fuel in the external tank is exhausted, the tank is jettisoned. The shuttle is now outside the gravitational pull of the earth and the shuttle's powered flight has ended. The spacecraft no longer requires those tremendous forces to propel it forward. It now uses small on-board thrusters to make simple course corrections, to explore and navigate its way in space. Without these simple course corrections, the orbit would quickly deteriorate and the shuttle would re-enter the earth's atmosphere somewhere over the Pacific Ocean. Similarly, at this point in the lean transformation, maintenance requires only simple efforts to hold the course. The organization must hold the course, however, and never become complacent. Without these simple course corrections, the lean transformation deteriorates and all the advances will be lost. A lean transformation is never complete. The lean culture developed during the transformation must be maintained and allowed to flourish.

Commitment, tenacity, and determination are the forces necessary to effectively break free of the pull to gravitate back to the existing system. Once a lean program is successfully launched, resistance to change will diminish. Momentum will increase and drive the transformation forward. Once the organization can consider itself a lean enterprise, only small corrections will be required to stay the course. Success lies in the hands of the hospital leadership and their commitment to the lean transformation.

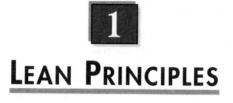

LEAN PRINCIPLES

Imagine yourself a patient coming to the Emergency Department at a local area hospital. You have pneumonia and will eventually be admitted, but at this time you have not yet been diagnosed. Upon entering the Emergency Department, you look around and see people who seem to be in much greater need of immediate attention than you. You walk up to the reception desk, give your name, describe your symptoms, and request to see a doctor. The receptionist instructs you to have a seat and wait to be called. A process has just begun that will last, on average, ten hours and fifty-one minutes (based on studies conducted by this author at several hospitals).

During these ten hours and fifty-one minutes, you will be examined, x-rays will be taken, and test specimens will be obtained and sent off for analysis. These process steps, all very important, will directly contribute to making you well. Surprisingly, the same studies show that the time required to complete these vital process steps accounts for less than ten percent of the ten hours and fifty-one minutes you will be in the Emergency Department. Other steps are necessary or required in order for care to be delivered safely and accurately, but these additional steps do not contribute to making you well. Once again, you will probably be surprised to learn that these process steps make up less than seven percent of the total process time. The remaining steps, which make up almost eighty-five percent of the total process time, are spent performing tasks that are neither required nor necessary and that do not contribute to making you well. Most of this time is spent waiting, clarifying, searching, transporting, and verifying. As a result, clinician's duties deviate from patient care and become administrative in nature. Dr. John Kenagy, a vascular surgeon turned efficiency expert, was quoted in Forbes magazine as saying that "nurses spend a third of their time in patient care and two thirds of their time hunting, documenting and clarifying" (Fisher, 2000). The elimination of operations that fall into these categories, neither required nor necessary and not contributing to making you well, is the basic concept behind Lean.

A HISTORY OF LEAN AND THE TOYOTA PRODUCTION SYSTEM

Established in April of 1950, Toyota Motor Sales Company, Ltd., launched a business during an era that should have resulted in failure. This was post-World War II Japan. The country was attempting to recover from the devastating effects of the bombing of many of its cities, including the incredibly destructive atomic bombings of Hiroshima and Nagasaki (Wikipedia, 2005). The basic necessities of life such as food, shelter, and natural resources were scarce or non-existent. In an effort to create economic growth, the country began to manufacture inexpensive consumer goods, classified by the rest of the world as junk, that earned the Japanese people a reputation for shoddy workmanship. The management at Toyota, however, understood that in order to gain recognition in the global marketplace they would need to provide a high-quality product at a competitive price. They also recognized that in order to accomplish this they would need to do more with less. This realization sparked the birth of the Toyota Production System (TPS), which today is more commonly known as lean manufacturing.

The basic underlying concept of TPS was to eliminate any operations that did not add value to the company's product or service from the standpoint of the final customer. The management at Toyota implemented this concept in every operation throughout their plant. They eliminated or minimized the need for their assemblers to walk, bend, reach, or turn. They implemented devices that eliminated mistakes or brought attention to mistakes before they became defects. They reduced inventories by providing the parts to the assembly lines "just in time" (JIT) instead of stockpiling huge quantities of parts "just in case" they were needed to complete an order. By eliminating delays and the constraints that caused these delays, TPS assured the continuous flow of the product from the beginning to the end of the process. Toyota's leaders eliminated the need to transport parts to different areas of the manufacturing floor and streamlined operations so that each step provided only what was needed when it was needed in the quantity it was needed every time it was needed. They developed new procedures for changing over from one product to another, which minimized machine downtime. The employees practiced these procedures so they could execute them correctly and safely in the least amount of time. In addition to implementing efficiency improvements, they also kept a close eye on quality by implementing statistical process control methods and empowering employees to react to problems. All employees who worked in the plant had the authority to stop the production line if they spotted a defect. This action would summon the immediate attention of management and engineering to quickly eliminate the problem and get the line back to producing defect-free products. Implementing these concepts allowed Toyota to provide a quality product at a competitive price.

The Toyota Corolla gained popularity in the United States during the 1973 OPEC oil embargo. Americans purchased the Corolla because it offered an alternative to the gas-guzzling American cars, but quickly noticed that the Corolla was also extremely reliable, less prone to breakdown, and subject to few, if any, defects. Although it was fuel efficiency that initially prompted people to purchase the Toyota, it was the auto maker's attention to quality that kept customers coming back and caused them to spread the word. Today, the Toyota Corolla is the best-selling automobile in the world. Toyota Motor Sales Company, Ltd. is the second-largest automobile manufacturer in the world and is slowly nudging General Motors out of the number one position, which it has held since 1931.

Lean manufacturing, derived from the Toyota Production System, has evolved over the past fifty years. Manufacturing and service organizations all over the world have successfully implemented these principles and are reaping enormous benefits. Lean principles are now being effectively implemented in hospitals with great success. The opportunities for lean in the healthcare environment are limitless. Implementation requires a new way of looking at the care delivery process, a paradigm shift, which will transform the way value is delivered to the patient/customer. To achieve a lean transformation, it's essential to thoroughly understand lean principles and lean tools and their application in a healthcare environment. This book provides all of these elements. It may be used as an implementation guide for initiating a lean transformation.

CATEGORIZING OPERATIONS

All operations within a process can be categorized in one of three ways. An operation or process step that contributes directly to providing the product or service the patient/customer desires is categorized as value-added. The definition of value is related to the customer and the service being provided. For example, when a doctor sends a patient to the hospital for tests, the patient may see value from the standpoint of having the test done as quickly and accurately as possible. The doctor is also a customer. To the doctor, value may mean seeing the test results the same day. A nurse on an inpatient unit is the customer of the Facilities Support department. To that nurse, value may mean having a leak under the medication room sink repaired quickly, permanently, and with as little effort on his or her part as possible. Identifying the customer and defining value from the standpoint of that customer is the first step in a lean transformation (Womack and Jones, 1996).

The next category includes process steps that do not contribute directly to providing the product or service the patient/customer desires but that are required or necessary. These operations are categorized as business-value-added because they add value only from the standpoint of the business, not the customer. These process steps may be the result of having to follow hospital policy, established procedures, or regulatory guidelines; they are often inherently inefficient. Lean makes every effort to minimize the time spent conducting business-value-added operations and, if possible, to eliminate them altogether.

The final category involves process steps that do not contribute directly to providing the product or service that the patient/customer desires and that are not required or necessary. These operations are categorized as non-value-added, and every effort should be made to eliminate them. Creating a process devoid of non-value-adding operations is the ultimate goal of lean.

WORKING VS. ADDING VALUE

The supposition is often made that if people are working, they are adding value. The Emergency Department example proves this to be false. Anyone can walk into an Emergency Department, in any hospital, anywhere, at almost anytime of the day, and witness a torrent of activity that involves staff members working harder and more diligently than is required by practically any other profession. Most of this work, however, is directed toward forcing an outdated and complex care delivery system to flow. Constraints inherent in the care delivery process cause delays in providing care. This, in turn, increases the actual workload on staff members.

Attempts to create movement in the care delivery process often result in frustration and exasperation because constraints exist at a point in the process beyond the limits of the department's control. This scenario is true not only for the Emergency Department (ED) but for every department in the hospital: Surgery, Diagnostic Imaging, Maternity Services, Inpatient Units, Laboratory, Pharmacy, even the Store Room. If the process does not flow, it is usually the result of one or more bottlenecks further downstream in the process. These constraints cause backups in upstream processes and create additional work for the staff of those upstream departments. A patient or product will move through a process only as quickly as allowed by the biggest constraint. For example, if a patient is ready to be moved from the ED to an inpatient unit where a bed is not available, the patient must remain in the ED. This patient must be cared for, re-evaluated regularly, medicated, fed, and kept informed of admission status. In addition, this patient occupies a room that could be utilized for the care of another patient. This, in turn, leads to longer patient wait times and overcrowding. The Inpatient Unit also experiences frustration in the effort to make a bed available. Downstream constraints they must deal with include staffing issues, problems with discharge planning, obtaining doctor's orders, and getting the Environmental Services department to assign someone to clean the room. Further complicating matters is the frustrated and extremely annoyed ED staff member calling every fifteen minutes to find out when the room will be ready.

The point to be taken from all of this is that everyone is working hard, dealing with real problems, trying to solve them as quickly as possible. Staff are stressed, frustrated, and doing their very best, but they are not adding value. Instead, they are trying to force a complex, outdated system to run smoothly so that they can do the job for which they studied, trained, and were hired to do, making patients well.

Only by analyzing the entire process, and identifying and eliminating all constraints, can hospitals transform the care delivery system.

BECOMING LEAN

A lean transformation involves improving the way value is delivered to the patient/customer. It entails the elimination of non-value-added activities and the reduction of time spent performing business-value-added operations. To accomplish this, it is necessary to expose these non-value-added activities and take immediate action to eliminate them. The tools described in this book were developed for just that purpose.

An organization does not become lean overnight. It takes years of hard work and persistence. A lean transformation requires top-down commitment combined with bottom-up implementation. It involves crossing departmental boundaries. The commitment of senior administration is by far the most critical requirement for the success of a lean transformation. This means active commitment, doggedly supporting the development of a lean culture, making Lean a standard agenda topic at organizational meetings, being vocal about the importance of Lean to the organization, and being visible in the support of lean initiatives. Without the commitment of senior administration, the lean transformation is destined for failure. Commitment can not be delegated. It is the sole responsibility of senior administration to lead the organizational culture change that is integral to the successful lean transformation. This does not mean that senior administrators must participate in lean initiatives such as 5S events or even approve all lean projects. Their time is much better spent running the hospital. They must however, understand the concepts and tools of lean and their application in the healthcare environment so that they can communicate intelligently regarding the lean transformation.

Communication and training are essential to the lean transformation. It is important that lean principles be understood by all members of the organization so that the purposes of lean initiatives are not misconstrued. This can only be accomplished through training at all levels of the organization. In addition to training, communicating successes heightens interest and stifles negativity. Lean is implemented from the bottom up. The people who do the work apply the tools and make the changes. It is important that these individuals know that successful implementation will not have a negative impact on themselves or on their coworkers.

The purpose of lean is to eliminate or minimize non-value-added process steps, not to eliminate jobs. The term *lean* may conjure up images of a butcher trimming the fat from a cut of beef to produce a nice thick steak. Consequently, many people interpret a lean organization as one that "trims the fat" by cutting jobs. In fact, there are real-life examples of lean consultants who have reengineered an organization's workplace resulting in significant job cuts. In contrast to this approach, a skilled and experienced lean consultant possesses the basic understanding that lean requires bottom-up implementation and recognizes that a workforce reduction strategy would be self defeating because workers are naturally reluctant to improve themselves out of a job. They will instead resist all efforts on the part of the organization to implement lean concepts.

Many organizations involved in a lean transformation have implemented "no layoff" policies that support the genuine purpose of the lean transformation. This type of policy does not restrict the organization from terminating individuals for poor performance or other legitimate reasons. Instead, it provides the security that staff members will not lose jobs as a result of a lean implementation project.

Lastly, the delivery of a product or service almost always requires crossing departmental lines. Management and staff may no longer view a process from a departmental perspective but must instead look at the entire value stream. This value stream comprises all the steps necessary to provide the patient/customer with the desired product or service. Most constraints to the flow of a process occur when departmental lines are crossed. Taking a value-stream perspective highlights these bottlenecks and forces resolution so that the product or service can be provided without interruption. To accomplish this, silos and departmental walls must be torn down and the needs and desires of the customer/patient must take precedence. Management and staff must become less territorial in their efforts to care for patients. Administrators must recognize that cooperation between departments is necessary to eliminate these issues.

PREREQUISITE TO LAUNCHING THE LEAN INITIATIVE

Before making any formal announcements, senior administrators must be comfortable with their commitment to a lean transformation and they must have a comprehensive understanding of lean principles. Without this commitment on the part of all senior staff members, the lean transformation will never come to fruition.

Implementation of the lean transformation should be linked to the organization's strategic plan. For this reason, a clear and concise strategic plan should exist and must include both short- and long-term goals for the hospital. Proper deployment of the strategic plan will ensure that everyone in the organization has a set of measurable, realistic goals for which, it is clearly understood, they will be held accountable. Linkage to the strategic plan is only one of the criteria that should be incorporated in project selection, but it is vital to the success of the overall lean transformation.

Only at this juncture should there be a formal announcement by senior administration that the organization has chosen to undergo a lean transformation. In conjunction with this announcement, training should be provided to introduce hospital staff to the lean concept and explain the importance of their support relative to this initiative.

Commitment on the part of senior administration, linkage to the organization's strategic plan, and the introduction of lean concepts to staff members provides a solid foundation from which to launch the lean transformation. It is now time for action.

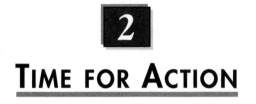

TIME FOR ACTION

The now famous Institute of Medicine (IOM) report *To Err Is Human: Building A Safer Medical System*, which estimated that preventable medical errors kill as many as 98,000 patients annually, has highlighted the inadequacies in the care delivery process. The report, however, does not attribute these errors to recklessness or incompetence on the part of caregivers, but rather to the complexity of the care delivery process (Committee on Quality of Healthcare in America, Institute of Medicine, 2000). With all the technological and scientific advances that have occurred in healthcare, it is amazing that changes in the care delivery system have been relatively nonexistent. In an article entitled *Healthcare's Need for Revolutionary Change*, Martin D. Merry, M.D., is quoted as saying, "Healthcare is now a $1.5 trillion industry–the largest of our society–built essentially around a craft model still rooted not in the twentieth or even the nineteenth century, but in the eighteenth" (Merry, 2003). The time for action is now. Hospitals must re-evaluate the care delivery system and create a new model devoid of non-value-added steps, user-friendly, free of constraints, and providing high-quality care to the patient/customer.

THE NEED FOR CHANGE

The need for change in healthcare has never been more apparent than it is today. Healthcare is the country's largest industry. It is poised for exponential growth as baby boomers reach their sixties, yet external influences make it more and more difficult for hospitals to prosper. Reimbursements are stagnant or declining as insurance companies and Medicare dictate prices. The number of uninsured people is on the rise. The Healthcare Financial Management Association (HFMA) estimates that 45 million Americans currently lack health insurance and this number is only expected to grow (2005). The demand for new physicians is growing more rapidly than the supply of practicing physicians is expected to grow. The Council on Graduate Medical Education predicts that the nation is likely to experience a shortage of 85,000 to 96,000 physicians by 2020 (2005). The Health Resources and Services Administration predicts that the national nursing shortage will top 800,000 by 2020 (2002). Other staff shortages are also expected, including Nuclear Medicine Technologist, MRI Technologist, Ultrasound Technologist, and Physician Assistant. The Blue Cross and Blue Shield Association points out that pharmaceuticals are the leading contributor to skyrocketing healthcare costs accounting for approximately 20 percent of overall costs, according to several sources they have surveyed (2004). The National Coalition on Health Care estimates that healthcare spending is 430 percent higher than what the nation spends on national defense (2004). Other contributors to rising healthcare costs include malpractice insurance, technological advances, and medical supplies. These factors have led to a weakened financial position and credit downgrades for many hospitals as their financial situations deteriorate. A growing number of our nation's hospitals are being forced to close their doors. There is a saying that some people take action when they see the light, others when they feel the heat. Too many hospitals are beginning to feel the heat. Like Toyota, they must take action and learn to do more with less. Lean has the very real potential to update the care delivery process to one that flows, error free, and delivers value from the standpoint of the patient/customer. There is, however, no time to waste. The time for action is now.

PREPARING FOR THE LEAN TRANSFORMATION

The decision to undergo a lean transformation is not one to be taken lightly. Lean is serious business that demands hard work, a major culture change, and a long-term commitment. It is not an initiative to be implemented halfheartedly. These statements are not meant to discourage hospital administrators considering a lean transformation, but rather to enlighten them. Nothing extraordinary comes without serious effort and commitment. Lean is not for short-sighted administrators looking for quick fixes that require minimal effort. On the contrary, lean requires strong leadership, visibility, and "walking the talk."

Don't be fooled by the implied simplicity of lean concepts, which are often equated with common sense. In reality, many of these concepts are counterintuitive and are extremely difficult to implement. Only with the experience gained through experimentation will staff members begin to apply lean principles and move the organization forward. Lean is not a "flavor of the month" initiative. It has been around for more than fifty years and has allowed companies to prosper through difficult times. Some organizations have failed in their lean transformation efforts, but regardless of the cynicism toward lean generated by these organizations, it was not the principles of lean that failed. These failures were more likely the result of a lackadaisical approach to the lean transformation, improper launch of the initiative, poor application of lean tools, or a combination of these factors. To avoid these pitfalls, careful planning of the initiative is critical to success.

Neither is lean a concept that can be implemented on an experimental basis for a week, a month, or even a year. A long-term commitment is required right from the start. Five years is a common and realistic timeframe in which to carry out a lean transformation. The rationale for requiring a five-year commitment is that lean transformation involves changing organizational culture. This means that all individuals in the organization must learn to look at the care delivery system differently. They must be taught the concepts of lean, be able to identify non-value-added operations, and be empowered to take action to eliminate them. Managers must support and teach rather than delegating work assignments and directing activities. Departmental walls must be torn down and departments must learn to work together from an organizational value-stream perspective. Accomplishing these things involves knowledge, understanding, tenacity, and experience acquired over time. Cutting corners is not acceptable. It is not realistic for an organization to assume that conducting twice as many lean events will lessen the time commitment. A lean transformation takes time and requires patience.

Quitting is not an option. Once the commitment has been made to move forward with lean, it is important to stick with it. At times it may seem as though the organization is moving backward. An axiom in lean points out that two steps forward and one step back is acceptable progress, but no steps forward and no steps back is not acceptable. Anyone who has experienced real sustained change knows that it takes time. Transformation is sometimes so gradual that it goes unnoticed, but the indicators of change are undeniable. Watching a lean transformation is analogous to watching a child grow. Every day the child grows in some way, but so gradually that it goes virtually unnoticed by the parents. When friends and relatives see the child, they will most certainly comment on how much he or she has grown. The indicators of growth are always present. Birthdays, graduations, and increasing independence are all proof positive that growth is taking place. Similarly, organizational change may not be immediately obvious, but increased revenue, reduced costs, greater patient satisfaction, and improved recruitment and retention are growth indicators that demonstrate advancement toward a lean enterprise. Those not directly associated with the organization on a daily basis will notice the change and comment on it.

Planning for lean transformation must be synchronized with the strategic plans for the hospital. If a strategic plan does not exist, one must be created. Hospital leadership must provide a clear and concise vision of where the organization wants to be in one, five, ten, and twenty years, in detail, along with a plan detailing the steps necessary to achieve these goals. Creating statements for mission, vision, and values is important, but without an action plan these statements are merely dreams.

Top-down deployment of the strategic plan is also essential. A strategic plan buried in a desk drawer or collecting dust on an office shelf is not much better than no plan at all. The purpose of a strategic plan is to breathe new life into an organization. All players must understand, and be held accountable for, their responsibilities in its execution. People generally perform better if they know what is expected of them. Goals must include the five necessary SMART attributes: Specific, Measurable, Attainable, Relevant, and Time bound. These five attributes ensure a thorough understanding of what is expected and provide criteria to denote successful achievement of the goal.

Once the groundwork has been completed, a formal announcement is made to everyone in the organization that the hospital is launching an initiative to become a lean organization. It must be made clear that lean is not just another program but rather a means to change the care delivery process and, more specifically, the value delivery process. Lean will be a way of life for the organization and its employees from this point on.

The formal announcement must be made by the CEO with all of his or her direct reports present. If one of them is sick, out of town, or unavailable for any reason, postpone the announcement until everyone is available. It is essential to show a united front and demonstrate commitment and buy-in from all the leaders of the organization. If possible, the presence of board members will help emphasize the organization's level of commitment. Begin the announcement by describing the obstacles influencing healthcare: declining reimbursements, high cost of technology, diminishing labor market, deteriorating financial situation, declining quality, increasing costs, and so on. Present these problems so they are easy to understand, provide as much detail as necessary to make them real, but be careful not to lose your audience with unnecessary facts. The goal is to "establish a sense of urgency" (Kotter, 1996), capturing everyone's attention and insuring that they understand the seriousness of the situation. A sense of urgency will motivate people to change. Next present the organization's strategy for dealing with these issues, outlining the plan to increase revenue, reduce costs, and improve quality. The strategy section should culminate with an explanation of the need for structural, procedural, and cultural change and the announcement that in order to accomplish this level of change the organization has made the commitment to a lean transformation. Most people won't know what it means to undergo a lean transformation, but this is not the time to provide training on lean principles, tools, and techniques. Instead, inform everyone that they will be scheduled to participate in a training session that will explain lean concepts and address any questions they may have. Reiterate the organization's commitment, stressing that the road ahead will be difficult and that time, patience, and persistence are essential to success.

All employees need to know that each and every one of them is integral to the success on this undertaking and that lean is not a staff reduction strategy. Lean is a growth strategy, a survival strategy, and an improvement strategy. The goal of lean is, first and foremost, to provide value to the patient/customer and, in so doing, eliminate the delays, overcrowding, frustration, irritation, and patient complaints associated with the existing system. Lean creates a better working environment where what is supposed to happen does happen, on time, every time. It allows clinicians to spend more of their time caring for patients and improves the quality of care these patients receive. A lean organization values its employees and encourages their involvement in organizational initiatives. This, in turn, sustains hospital-wide quality improvements. The first step to achieving a successful lean transformation and becoming a lean hospital involves the careful preparation outlined in this section. Do not skip any of these steps or assume they can be done at a later date. This will only create the illusion of forward momentum and will result in a setback later in the transformation process.

PROJECT SELECTION

Once the formal announcement has been made and everyone has attended an overview session outlining the underlying principles of lean, it is time to implement. By this time, everyone will be anxious to see lean in action and to evaluate for themselves the results of the first lean improvement event. For this reason it is most important to start with one or two projects that have a high likelihood of success and that will provide a big payback. This need not be the deciding factor in project selection going forward, but it is highly recommended in the early stages of launching the initiative.

A decision matrix is an effective tool for selecting projects. It is based on criteria established by senior administration, with each criterion assigned a weight relative to the overall objective. At a minimum, the criteria should include linkage to the strategic plan, expected payback, level of effort required, risk involved, likelihood of success, and impact for the customer/patient.

The steps for creating a decision matrix are covered in detail in Chapter 6, and an example of a decision matrix for project selection is provided in Figure 2.1. Each criterion becomes a column heading; each row is dedicated to a proposed project. Projects are evaluated relative to each criterion and given a score based on the assigned scoring values. Scores are multiplied by the weight factor and summed at the end of each row. In most cases, the project with the highest score should be selected for implementation.

The example shown in Figure 2.1 indicates that likelihood of success is the major factor in project selection and carries a weight factor of 2. Future projects may weight each criterion differently based on what the organization is trying to accomplish. Administrators decide what weight to assign each category depending on the objective.

Project Selection Matrix

	Linkage to strategic plan	Level of effort required	Risk involved	Likelihood of success	Impact for customer	Expected payback	Total
	1 – Low 3 – Mid Range 9 – High	1 – Difficult 3 – Reasonable 9 – Easy	1 – High 3 – Some 9 – Low	1 – Poor 3 – Good 9 – Excellent	1 – Low 3 – Mid Range 9 – High	1 – Low 3 – Mid Range 9 – High	
Weight	1	1.5	0.5	2	1	1.5	
Project 1	9	3	1	3	3	1	27.5
Project 2	3	9	3	9	1	1	39.5
Project 3	1	1	3	1	3	3	16.5

FIGURE 2.1 Project-selection matrix, demonstrating weighting criteria based on organizational objectives.

Once the project has been selected, it is time to schedule and conduct the lean event. It is recommended to focus on one event at a time in the early stages of the lean transformation. As the organization becomes more proficient with lean tools and concepts, multiple events can be scheduled and conducted simultaneously. Follow the steps for conducting a lean event outlined in Chapter 8. Upon completion of the event, post an open invitation to all employees to attend the final presentation. If necessary, conduct more than one presentation so everyone interested has the opportunity to attend. It is important, especially in the early stages of a lean transformation, to provide everyone the opportunity to see what can be accomplished by implementing lean concepts. Individuals in the organization will be evaluating the soundness of the initiative and will be conducting a mental assessment regarding what they see, hear, and experience relative to the transformation.

Ultimately, individuals will accept or reject lean principles based on the information they collect. They will want to know how becoming a lean hospital will benefit them ("What's in it for me?"). As they begin this mental assessment they may assume, based on past experience with other programs, that lean will mean more work, more responsibility, and greater time commitment. They may even have concerns related to job security resulting from rumors from other organizations. It is critical that everyone see clearly that lean principles lead to less time spent conducting non-value-added process steps, more time involved in patient care, happier patients, and fewer problems. Lean will also reduce costs and increase revenues, thereby enhancing job security.

THE DECISION TO HIRE A CONSULTANT

Although the application of lean tools appears to be common sense, the concepts may be difficult to implement until an adequate knowledge base is formed and sufficient experience is acquired. Lean implementation is not something one can learn in a classroom, from a video, or by reading a book. The only way to learn how to implement lean is by doing it. A hospital just starting out on its lean journey is well advised to employ the services of a consultant or to hire someone with lean implementation experience to head up the lean transformation initiative. Whichever path the organization chooses, be sure to find someone with experience implementing lean concepts in hospitals.

Almost all lean consulting firms, and there are many, will claim to be experts in lean implementation. Some are, but many more are not. Regardless of an individual's knowledge and familiarity with lean, experience in a hospital environment is essential for success.

Some firms will try to convince you that healthcare is no different from manufacturing. Although it is true that the same techniques are employed across both industries, there are major differences between the two. The two most significant differences are inventory and repetition. Manufacturing companies have huge sums of money tied up in work-in-process inventory and parts. A consultant in that environment has the opportunity to implement one-piece flow rather easily, quickly cutting inventory levels by fifty percent or more and saving the company considerable money. Hospitals do not afford this opportunity because very little of their assets are tied up in work-in-process inventory. A consultant with only manufacturing experience would not be able to apply the same lean concepts and reap the same benefits.

The other significant difference between hospitals and manufacturing plants is that almost all the work performed in a manufacturing plant is repetitious. A worker on the manufacturing floor will conduct the same task or series of tasks the same way, over and over, throughout the course of a day, a week, a month, or even a year. This is not true in healthcare. It would make life much easier for healthcare workers if pneumonia patients were only admitted on Mondays, patients with congestive heart failure were cared for on Tuesdays, and emergency surgeries were only performed on the third Thursday of each month. This is not the case in healthcare and hospital staff members must deal with whatever comes their way. An experienced healthcare consultant could adapt the lean concepts in hospital-specific situations.

Reimbursements based on diagnosis codes, the high costs associated with pharmaceuticals, the rising number of uninsured patients, and staffing shortages are just some of the other issues associated with healthcare. A lean consultant with only manufacturing experience would be unfamiliar with these issues.

Yet another benefit to finding a consultant with experience in healthcare is his or her access to other hospitals engaged in lean transformation. This access and knowledge sharing can save considerable time, money, and grief in the implementation process.

Whether a hospital chooses to hire a lean healthcare consultant or not, serious consideration should be given to the appointment of a lean leader. The lean leader will work closely with the consultant or the person heading up the lean transformation to put in place a plan to transfer knowledge and experience to the lean leader. Once the lean leader has sufficient experience, the services of a consultant can be significantly reduced and eventually eliminated completely.

In the early stages of a lean transformation, the services of a consultant may be required only once every four to six weeks. This should taper down to once a quarter after nine to twelve months. A healthcare consultant's primary responsibility is to provide guidance for the organization in its lean transformation. The transfer of knowledge to the hospital staff and the development of a lean mentality are the primary reasons for employing the services of a lean consultant. The goal is not to provide steady employment for the consultant but rather for the organization to become self sufficient in its ability to become a lean enterprise.

As the person responsible for heading up the lean transformation and facilitating lean events, the lean leader should be a direct report to the hospital president. The president has ultimate responsibility for the lean transformation and requires first-hand knowledge regarding progress, obstacles, and resistance to the initiative. Filtering this information through a chain of command could result in false, ambiguous, or distorted communication. The lean leader must be able to convey all communication directly to the president of the hospital.

THE TRANSFORMATION PROCESS

Up to this point the organization has done much preparation and training and conducted the first lean event. There may have been some celebrating to mark the hospital's official entry into the lean journey ahead. What now?

The lean transformation consists of a series of lean events. Each event should last three to five days and requires a bias for getting things done. The Japanese call it *kaikaku*, or radical improvement. These events are often selected based on the need established during the value-stream mapping process. The future state value stream map (see Chapter 4) will highlight and provide the valuable information related to areas that are constraints to flow. However, the value-stream map is not the only method for identifying opportunities for improvement. Using a decision matrix, administration can prioritize and select the lean events to be conducted and the order in which they are to be executed. Regardless of what method is used to choose and prioritize events, be sure there is tie-in to the hospital's strategic plan.

A lean event should be scheduled every month in order to generate and maintain momentum. If resources pose a serious issue relative to organizing an improvement team, it is acceptable to conduct an event every six weeks. The staff must see that hospital administrators are committed to the lean transformation and they must see progress. Too much time between events can cause momentum and enthusiasm to wane. Four-week intervals are optimum, especially during the early stages of implementation.

Once an event is completed, put that same project on the schedule to be revisited in eight to twelve months. Having conducted an event does not mean that all the opportunities to eliminate non-value-added operations, to create flow, or to improve the process have been exhausted. Remember, there's always room for improvement. Even if all opportunities for improvement were exhausted, things change. New methods are introduced, new equipment is purchased, regulations change, and so on. Change is inevitable. In the words of Heraclitus of Ephesus, "nothing endures but change, change is the only constant."

Conduct lean events, as outlined in Chapter 8, by implementing the tools introduced in this book. This is not an all-inclusive listing of the tools of lean. These are, however, the basic and fundamental tools that your organization needs to begin and sustain a lean transformation. Beyond the lean tools presented in this book, a few others will be necessary prior to the later stages of the lean transformation. For more information about other tools available in the lean toolbox, refer to the glossary at the end of this book.

A LEAN ROAD MAP

A lean transformation is a serious undertaking requiring commitment, time, patience, tenacity, and a willingness to change. This chapter defines a series of steps which, if adhered to, will insure that the lean journey will end at the desired destination. Arbitrarily conducting lean events to resolve issues that arise in the normal course of conducting business may alleviate a current problem but will not get the organization any closer to its destination. As with a road trip, the lean journey must first identify the destination, lay out the route, divide the trip into segments, and travel the necessary distance to complete each segment. As with any road trip, there will be bumps in the road and detours along the way. Be prepared for these anomalies so as to minimize the impact.

KNOW YOUR DESTINATION

Knowing the destination is the first step on the road to a lean organization. This may seem obvious. One wouldn't get into a car or any other vehicle without knowing the final destination, yet many organizations embark on a journey to change an entire organization without a clear destination in mind. Ultimately the goal is to increase revenue, reduce cost, and improve quality, but these goals are not specific enough.

Vision statements were popular in the 1990s. Many organizations developed statements of mission (what is the organization's business?), vision (what does the organization want to be?) and values (what are the priorities in the organization's culture?). Administrators spent months, sometimes years, developing these statements. Today these expensive frames and laminated hardwood plaques hang on walls as reminders of a different era. These statements must be taken down, dusted off, updated as necessary, and acted upon, especially the vision statement. Everyone in the organization should know the vision and his or her role in achieving it.

Once the vision is clearly established, a detailed plan is required to make the vision a reality. The development of a strategic plan should begin with an analysis of the current situation, commonly referred to as a SWOT analysis. What are the organization's strengths, weaknesses, opportunities, and threats? Strengths and weaknesses are internal factors affecting the organization such as capabilities and competencies. Opportunities and threats relate to external factors such as environment and competitive edge. With a viable and realistic strategic plan in place, the organization will become more proactive than reactive in bringing its vision to fruition, giving it greater control over its own destiny.

A strategic plan by itself is merely a document. The plan must be executed in order to obtain the desired results. Everyone in the hospital must understand his or her role in helping the organization achieve its strategic initiative. This is accomplished through strategy deployment.

STRATEGY DEPLOYMENT

In many organizations the strategic plan never moves to the next level; it remains simply a plan. Directors and managers are never made to understand their roles in the overall plan for the hospital. They continue to plan their own strategies at an operational level. Without strategy deployment, how will people know what they are responsible for relative to organizational growth? How will they be held accountable when the organization's vision fails to materialize?

Strategic deployment involves a series of cascading strategy deployment sessions conducted annually. These sessions begin with the CEO and his or her direct reports and continue through the organization to whatever level seems appropriate. Based on the strategic plan, four to eight areas of strategic focus are established. Areas of strategic focus might include improved patient satisfaction, reduced medical errors, or finance. Under each area of strategic focus, goals are established for each individual participating in the session. These goals become more detailed as the sessions cascade through the organization.

Strategic deployment ensures that everyone knows what is required, when goals must be accomplished, and how performance will be evaluated. Once these goals are established, individuals must be held accountable; they should be justly rewarded when goals are met.

THE VALUE STREAM

At this point, everyone should have a thorough understanding of what the organization is trying to achieve and what their roles are in realizing the hospital's vision. They should recognize that they can no longer operate on a departmental level. Instead, as part of a much bigger picture, they must act on improving the whole. To do this, it's necessary that everyone understand the concept of value stream. The value stream is everything that must occur in order to provide a service to the patient/customer. The value stream crosses departmental boundaries and is defined from a patient/customer perspective.

It's important to develop a value stream map for each area of strategic focus based on the goals developed during the strategic deployment sessions. For example, a long-term strategic initiative may be to create efficient patient flow through the Emergency Department. Assume that this initiative is categorized under the patient satisfaction area of strategic focus. In year one, a goal may be to identify the leading constraint(s) to patient flow, schedule and conduct lean events to address these constraints, and reduce overall wait times by 25 percent. By mapping the value stream (see Chapter 4: Value Stream Mapping), the hospital is able to see the existing constraints to flow, to identify non-value-added operations, and to visualize how the process should flow.

Each organization should generate two maps, the first depicting the way the process operates currently (Current State Map), and the second portraying the desired process (Future State Map).

DEVELOP A WORK PLAN

The completed value stream map, if done thoroughly and completely, may be overwhelming. Keep in mind that the value stream is the entire flow through the facility. It will encompass several departments and highlight many constraints to flow. Attempting to realize the complete future state model all at once would be impractical and, in all probability, impossible. Instead, the current state map is divided into subdivisions that will afford a more realistic and manageable approach to obtaining the desired goal. Examples of possible subdivisions might include:

- Diagnostic Imaging Subdivisions
    - Develop continuous flow through department
    - Reduce cycle times
    - Increase equipment uptimes
    - Develop a pull system for report
- Laboratory Services Subdivisions
    - Establish work cells
    - Implement one-piece flow for specimens
    - Reduce changeover time
- Inpatient Unit Subdivisions
    - Establish a pull system for beds
    - Reduce Average Length of Stay (ALOS)
    - Reduce room changeover time

The next step is to develop a value stream work plan (see Chapter 5: Value Stream Mapping). The value stream work plan is a Gantt chart, essential to project management. A value stream work plan establishes deadlines, identifies milestones, assigns resources, and defines prerequisites, thereby organizing and tracking the path to the future state.

CREATE FLOW

The ultimate goal of lean is to create flow and pull value through the value stream by eliminating operations that do not add value. There are three key elements to successful lean implementation:

1. Standard work

2. User-friendliness

3. Unobstructed throughput

STANDARD WORK

Standard work involves reducing process steps to a series of individual tasks devoid of non-value-added activity and executed in a specific sequence. The time required to complete each task is indicated and conducted in accordance with customer demand. Lean utilizes standard work forms in order to obtain necessary information for the development of standard work. These forms are introduced in Chapter 5: Standard Work. They are the Standard Work Sheet, Time Observations Sheet, Combination Sheet, and Percent Load Chart. These forms allow the team to assess the current process, identify areas of non-value-added activity, provide clarity relative to what type of action is necessary, and document the new standard work.

Properly formulated standard work provides high-quality care to the patient when it's needed, safely, efficiently, and without error. In order to execute standard work, the process must be user-friendly.

USER-FRIENDLINESS

User-friendliness means providing for the patient and/or staff what is needed, when it is needed, in the quantity it is needed, on time, every time, twenty four hours a day, seven days a week, three hundred and sixty five days a year. Standard work can be executed only if supplies are readily available, if medications are delivered to the unit on time, if equipment is in working order, if the process is clearly defined. The concept of standard work falls apart if supplies are unavailable, if the process includes workarounds or stop-gap measures, if additional instruction is required.

Imagine a NASCAR pit crew, highly skilled, coordinated, and proficient. In 18.5 seconds the pit crew changes all four tires, refuels the vehicle, cleans the windshield and grill, and sends the driver back onto the track. Standard work exists for the pit crew. The entire process is reduced to a series of individual tasks devoid of non-value-added operations. These tasks are executed in a pre-determined sequence within a specified time, all in accordance with customer demand. The driver receives high-quality workmanship when it's needed, without error, efficiently, and safely. Now imagine the same pit crew missing a jack, searching for a lug nut, trying to verify if the fuel in the container is the correct octane, and searching for a solvent that will get the bugs off the windshield. This driver is not likely to be back on the track in 18.5 seconds. In fact, with a pit crew as unorganized, confused, and inefficient as this, the driver may never make it back to the track. The most highly-skilled crew can not execute standard work if the process is not user-friendly. This is the same image that hospitals convey to their patients when the process is not user-friendly. The most competent, highly trained, and compassionate care giver will be viewed as unorganized, confused, and inefficient if the process is not user-friendly.

UNOBSTRUCTED THROUGHPUT

With standard work in place and a user-friendly process, the only additional requirement is to eliminate constraints to flow. A process can move only as quickly as its biggest constraint allows. Moving a constraint to another point within the value stream creates work in queue for process steps upstream from the constraint and inefficiencies for process steps downstream. There are three options for dealing with a constraint: eliminate it, target it for improvement to reduce its process time, or balance all processes upstream and downstream from the constraint in order to minimize or eliminate its effects. These options may be accomplished by conducting a series of lean events (see Chapter 9: Conducting a Lean Event) and implementing the tools described in this book.

The chapter on standard work introduces the forms and the methods needed to identify, time, sequence, and balance individual tasks within a process and to develop standard work. Kanban, 5S, Visual Controls, Mistake Proofing, Quick Changeover, and Six Sigma enhance standard work, make the process user-friendly, and provide unobstructed throughput. The chapter on conducting lean events steps the reader through a lean event from planning to final presentation. Events should be scheduled as often as possible, ideally once a month. These events typically last three to five days. Several events may be conducted during the same three- to five-day period.

PROCEED WITH CAUTION

It would be naive to believe that everyone in the organization will rally behind the lean transformation. In reality, many will resist any kind of change, especially in the initial stages of an initiative. Most will eventually come around, but be wary of those who do not.

- Resistance comes in many forms—from passive resistance to strong opposition. Immediately address resistance in any form, before it grows and spreads throughout the organization. Ignoring resistance can validate a reluctance to commit on the part of other staff members.

- People respond better to constructive comments. Reprimands and threats rarely work. Instead, they often cause people to stand firm and become even less flexible in their views. Communication, training, and persuasion are the preferred methods for dealing with resistance.

- If senior administrators do not take the initiative seriously, their direct reports won't take it seriously either.

- Always treat people with dignity. Everyone wants to feel important and everyone has something to offer. Lean requires bottom-up implementation. The people who do the work understand the processes better than anyone else. They almost always know the problems and often have the solutions. Someone should listen to them.

- Give people enough time to acclimate to the change initiative. To gain acceptance; communicate successes, reinforce commitment, and provide training.

- Having people participate in an event is key to gaining acceptance, but be wary of "anchor draggers." Anchor draggers are individuals who constantly reject change. They use expressions such as, "You can't change this" and "We've already tried that and it doesn't work." They add a "but" at the end of their sentences (that is, "Looks good on paper, but…," "That's all well and good, but…," "That sounds like a great idea, but…."). An anchor dragger can easily sabotage a lean event. Remove team members who constantly raise objections or in any way hinder progress and proceed without them.

LEAN ORGANIZATIONAL ROLES

Everyone in the hospital has responsibilities relative to the success of the lean transformation that are beyond those normally seen within an organization. In a lean hospital the organizational pyramid is inverted (see Figure 3.1). The President, the CEO, and senior administrators support the pyramid. They have a working knowledge of lean principles, they are vocal about the importance of lean to the organization and visible in support of lean initiatives, and they commit the resources necessary for success. Management, which includes directors, managers, supervisors, and team leaders, provides guidance for lean implementation. They understand lean principles and tools, lead lean events, develop the lean culture, and teach rather than direct. At the top of the inverted pyramid are the front-line staff members who participate in lean events, develop a heightened awareness for non-value-added process steps and, most importantly, follow standard work. Management must provide encouragement and guidance and empower staff to make improvements and eliminate non-value-added process steps.

Follow this road map to reach your destination of becoming a lean organization.

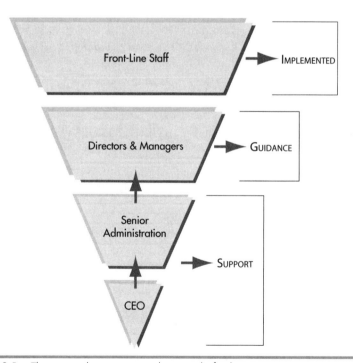

FIGURE 3.1   The inverted organizational pyramid of a lean organization.

4

VALUE STREAM MAPPING

Value stream mapping provides a high-level view of a process that has been targeted for improvement. Depending on the process being mapped, it may include the entire service line from patient presentation to discharge or from order to completion. The value stream illustrates both the physical flow of a patient or product through the organization and the information flow related to the patient or product. While process improvement efforts focus on the details of a specific process (for example, the individual steps associated with taking an x-ray), the value stream focus is on the entire process from beginning to end. The ability to focus on both of these areas is essential to the transformation of the value delivery process.

The Joint Commission for the Accreditation of Healthcare Organizations (JCAHO) requires hospitals to assess throughput and address the causes of constraints to patient flow throughout the organization. This standard (in the Hospital Leadership chapter, LD.3.15) states, "The leaders develop and implement plans to identify and mitigate impediments to efficient patient flow throughout the hospital" (2005). The Rationale for LD.3.15 includes the following statement:

"This standard emphasizes the role of assessment and planning for effective and efficient patient flow throughout the organization. To understand the system implications of the issues, leadership should identify all of the processes critical to patient flow through the hospital system from the time the patient arrives, through admitting, patient assessment and treatment, and discharge. Supporting processes such as diagnostic, communication, and patient transportation are included if identified by leadership as impacting patient flow. Relevant indicators are selected and data is collected and analyzed to enable monitoring and improvement of processes. (The Joint Commission for the Accreditation of Healthcare Organizations, 2005).

This is the essence of value stream mapping. As specified in the Rationale for LD.3.15, "leadership should identify all of the processes critical to patient flow through the hospital system from the time the patient arrives, through admitting, patient assessment and treatment, and discharge." (The Joint Commission for the Accreditation of Healthcare Organizations, 2005). This can be accomplished by drawing a value stream map for each product or service family. Value stream mapping not only highlights the constraints to flow but also exposes the non-value-added steps associated with the delivery of patient care.

Most organization-initiated process improvement efforts are restrained by process or departmental boundaries. As a result, these improvement initiatives take on a departmental perspective rather than a value stream perspective. By mapping the value stream, departmental boundaries are crossed and patient flow throughout the hospital can be clearly assessed from start to finish.

VALUE STREAM MAPPING DEFINED

Value stream mapping (VSM) uses symbols to create a map of the patient or product flow through the organization and the flow of information associated with the patient or product. The value stream map differs from a flow chart or process map in that it provides valuable information associated with the flow of the process.

VSM is a straightforward tool that does not require computers or sophisticated devices. A pencil and paper are all that is required to create a VSM. An organization may consider purchasing one of the many VSM software products on the market. These products may be useful for presentation purposes, but from the improvement perspective they add no value and may simply use up time that could be better spent improving the process. VSM is a simple yet powerful tool that should be kept simple. Even the use of a pen instead of a pencil may be objectionable. When mapping the value stream, especially early on, there will be many mistakes and correcting by erasure is much easier than starting anew. Remember, the goal is to highlight constraints and expose non-value-added steps, not to create a work of art.

DEFINITIONS

Before drawing a value stream map, it is important to know and understand how to determine and/or calculate key information. One must thoroughly understand the meaning of terms such as *Takt time, cycle time, flow, push, pull*, and others that are part of the lean organization's everyday vocabulary.

TAKT TIME

Takt is a German word referring to the baton used by an orchestra conductor. Just as the orchestra must keep pace with the conductor, the processes within the hospital must keep pace with patient/customer demand. Takt time is simple to calculate but somewhat confusing to understand. Dividing available time by patient/customer demand determines the pace of patient/customer demand and is the formula for calculating takt. If the organization provides a service for only one shift, the available time is 8 hours minus two 15-minute breaks, or 450 minutes. Accordingly, the available time for two shifts is 900 minutes; for three shifts it's 1350 minutes. Patient/customer demand is simply the number of times a particular service is performed on a daily basis. For example, each day a hospital may be required to perform 225 electrocardiograms (ECG), conduct 1800 urine analyses, and mix and deliver 450 IV Admixtures. The takt time for each of these services is calculated separately; it is dependent on the number of shifts dedicated to each service.

For illustrative purposes let us assign one shift to electrocardiograms, two shifts to urine analysis, and three shifts to IV Admixtures. The calculations for each of these three takt times (TT) is:

Electrocardiograms TT = 450 min. ÷ 225 ECG = 2 min. per ECG
Urine Analysis TT = 900 min. ÷ 1800 analysis = 30 sec. per analysis
IV Admixture TT = 1350 min. ÷ 450 mixtures = 3 min. per mixture

In order for the hospital to keep pace with patient/customer demand, it must perform one ECG every two minutes, a urine analysis every thirty seconds, and the mixing and delivery of one IV Admixture every three minutes.

To avoid confusion, remember that only two things can affect takt time: available time and patient/customer demand. Available time is directly proportional to takt time. If available time increases, TT will increase; if available time decreases, TT will decrease. Patient/customer demand is inversely proportional to takt time; it will have the opposite effect.

If two Cardio Pulmonary Techs are conducting electrocardiograms on the first shift in the example given, the takt time does not change. It is still 2 minutes per ECG. If two Lab Techs are performing urine analyses on first shift and one on second shift, the takt time does not change. It is still 30 seconds per analysis. If there are three Pharmacy Techs on each of the three shifts, the takt time is still 3 minutes per mixture. Regardless of the number of employees assigned to a task, the available time does not change and therefore the takt time does not change.

The same is true for lower staffing levels. If a hospital assigns only one Cardio Pulmonary Tech to do electrocardiograms for four hours a day, the takt time does not change. The hospital will not keep pace with demand, but the takt time does not change. This is a key point. The calculation of takt time has nothing to do with whether or not the hospital is keeping pace with demand. It has nothing to do with staffing levels or variation in the time needed to produce a product or perform a service. Takt time is simply the pace at which the product or service must be provided in order to meet patient/customer demand. Takt time is a goal. It tells management how to staff in order to keep pace with demand. It also tells management that a process must be targeted for improvement to reduce process times and meet takt time with the same staffing levels.

It may be necessary to recalculate takt time on a daily basis or even more than once a day. If demand is greater in the morning than the afternoon, it might be necessary to calculate a morning takt time and an afternoon takt time.

CYCLE TIME

Before cycle time can be thoroughly understood, it is important to differentiate between an operation and a process. A *process* is a series of tasks performed to provide a service or produce a product. An *operation* is each individual task that is performed within a process. Each operation falls into one of four categories: service, preparation, transportation, or queue. The *service* category includes the actual performance of the service being provided, such as taking an x-ray. *Preparation* includes all the things that must be done to prepare the patient and/or equipment to provide the service. Starting an IV or having the patient drink contrast for an x-ray fall into the preparation category. The third category, *transportation*, includes transporting the patient and/or materials to the site at which the service is to be performed. The last category is *queue*, which includes all the waiting time associated with performing the service. Everything done to provide a service falls into one of these four categories. Stringing together a series of operations creates a process, for example an outpatient visit to obtain a flu shot. Patients enter the hospital and provide their names and the reason for their visit to the receptionist (preparation). They are then instructed to have a seat and wait to be called (queue). Next, the patients walk to the designated area (transportation). The flu shot is administered (service) and the process is complete.

Cycle time is the amount of time necessary to complete one cycle of an operation or a process. Be sure to differentiate between operation cycle time and process cycle time, they are not interchangeable. Cycle time includes the value-added, business-value-added, and non-value-added steps within the operation or process.

FLOW

The concept of flow is simple. *Flow* is the continuous movement of process steps along the value stream. Flow is accomplished through the elimination of constraints or obstacles that impede the movement of the patient or product from one operation or process to the next. Creating flow is one of the major objectives of the lean transformation process. To create flow is to create a process that removes obstacles and minimizes preparation, transportation, and queuing operations, thereby delivering the service in the most efficient way possible. Flow may be interrupted whenever processes are disconnected or whenever it is necessary to cross departmental boundaries. Only by taking a value-stream perspective and evaluating the organization as a whole, rather than as individual departments or processes, can patient or product flow be accomplished.

PUSH

Push involves providing a product or service in anticipation of a need. It is always associated with high inventory in the form of products or patients. If the pharmacy is mixing drugs in anticipation of patient needs before orders are issued, they are pushing. If IVs are started on six patients awaiting nuclear stress tests, it is a push.

A problem associated with push, in addition to high inventory levels, is the propagation of errors and higher error rates. If an error occurs during the mixing of batches of drugs, the resulting defect will be present in all of the mixes in that batch. On the other hand, if only the needed drug were mixed and an error detected, only one product would be defective. Subsequent products would be defect free. Push is an intolerable method of providing a product or service; it must be eliminated and replaced with a pull system in order to accomplish flow.

PULL

Pull is a technique by which a product or service is provided only when a need arises. It is synonymous with the "Just In Time" philosophy—providing what is needed, when it's needed, in the quantity needed, on time, every time. Downstream processes pull from upstream processes. This means that processes occurring later in the value stream (downstream) pull from processes that occur earlier in the value stream (upstream). For example, consider the process for blood draw that involves registration followed by drawing the specimen. If the actual blood draw takes less time than registration, the phlebotomist will pull patients from registration. Conversely, if the actual blood draw takes longer than registration, the registrar will be pushing the patients to the blood draw station. Patients will accumulate in the waiting room while the phlebotomist tries to keep up with the push of patients. Replacing push with pull is essential to creating flow and a major phase in the lean transformation.

CHANGEOVER TIME

Changeover time is the time required to change over from one patient or product to the next. Changeover time begins when the current process of providing a product or service is finished and ends when the next product or service begins. Simply stated, it is the time between services when nothing is happening. For example, the changeover time for a CT-Scan is the elapsed time between the end of services to patient A, when the machine is turned off, and the time service begins for patient B, when the machine is turned on and the scan begins. Reducing changeover time can have a huge impact on throughput and significantly increase the efficiency of equipment.

At a minimum, the information provided for each process represented on the value stream map should include takt time, cycle time, and the number of employees assigned to the process. Changeover time should also be included, when applicable.

VSM SYMBOLS

The symbols used in value stream mapping are simple, commonsense representations of what they are designed to symbolize. Originally developed for manufacturing, these symbols may not lend themselves to healthcare processes. They may be easily altered or replaced by new symbols that make more sense for healthcare, if desired. The only hard and fast rule relative to symbols is uniformity. Decide on a set of symbols and use them consistently for all maps throughout the organization.

The first symbol is the process box. It is similar to the process box used in flowcharting, with the addition of a field across the top of the box in which is written the process name (see Figure 4.1). Information related to the process step is written in the area below the process name. This information includes but is not limited to takt time, cycle time, and the number of employees. The box may be enlarged to include additional information as required.

A new process box is needed whenever flow is interrupted or whenever processes are disengaged, but not for different operations within the same process. Remember, the value-stream map represents a high-level view of the process. As in flowcharting, the process boxes are connected by arrows. Unlike flowcharting, different arrows are used to connect the different boxes (see Figure 4.2). Transport and information arrows should include an information box indicating what is being transported or what information is being provided.

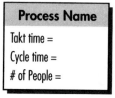

FIGURE 4.1 Process box.

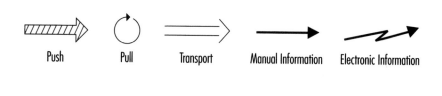

FIGURE 4.2 Examples of arrows used in value stream mapping.

The supplier of a patient, product, or service is depicted by means of a house-shaped box. Suppliers such as x-ray, laboratory, or M.D. office are identified inside the box. The database is represented by a cylinder, inventory by a triangle, and sequence of flow by the letters FIFO (First In First Out), LIFO (Last In First Out), or ACUITY (in the case of triage as with patients treated in the Emergency Department). Other symbols used in value-stream mapping include a kanban symbol, the flowchart symbol for a card, along with a dotted line showing the path of the kanban. Information symbols are simply a rectangle and areas targeted for improvement are represented by an explosion icon. Examples of all of these symbols are provided in Figure 4.3.

Value stream mapping involves the drawing of two maps, a current-state map and a future-state map. The current state map depicts the value stream as it exists now. It provides a baseline, exposes non-value-added steps, and highlights constraints to flow. The future state provides a picture of how the value stream would flow in a lean organization. The future state map represents the ideal state, a value stream devoid of non-value-added steps, free of constraints, and exceeding customer expectations. Once a plan is formulated and executed to achieve future state, this becomes the current state map and the process begins again.

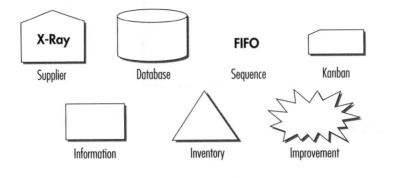

FIGURE 4.3   Basic flowcharting symbols employed in value stream mapping.

DRAWING A MAP OF THE CURRENT STATE

When drawing a value stream map it is important to focus on one product or service family and map it from beginning to end. If the intent is to map the flow of patients through the Emergency Department (ED), it is not necessary to map the flow of specimens taken from an ED patient through the Laboratory process. It is, however, necessary to indicate that the specimens are transported, orders are sent, and results are received. Mapping processes that take place in the Laboratory would make the map overly complicated since the Lab provides services for many other departments. If, however, the turnaround time for Laboratory test results is identified as a major bottleneck on the Emergency Department's current state map, then the use of an explosion icon would indicate the need to conduct a lean event in the Laboratory. In conjunction with this initiative, the flow of specimens through the Laboratory should be mapped as part of this separate improvement initiative.

To draw a value stream map you need only a pencil with an eraser and an 11″ x 17″ sheet of paper. Although not necessary, a stopwatch will definitely prove useful during the mapping process. Estimated cycle times are not reliable and should be used only when actual cycle times are too long to observe. Whenever possible, use a stopwatch or other timing mechanism to obtain cycle times by actual time observations.

Never map the value stream from memory. No matter how familiar you are with the process, go out to the floor and map the value stream by walking from one process step to the next, gathering the required information. Do not divide the process steps among team members and then try to piece it together later on. Segmenting the process steps means that none of the team members gets a clear picture of the overall value stream. The risk is that the handoffs and work arounds will not be identified. Draw the map as a team, with one person doing the actual drawing and the other team members providing inputs based on their individual observations.

Please refer to Appendix A for information on the process (blood draw) that will be utilized to demonstrate drawing a value stream map. The example used for this demonstration is the outpatient blood draw process of a fictitious hospital called University Hospital. The three processes associated with outpatient blood draw are reception, registration and phlebotomy. The department is open for one shift, during which the staff receives two 15-minute breaks. Because the department processes 100 patients a day, takt time can be calculated as follows:

$$\frac{(8 \text{ hours} * 60 \text{ min.}) - (2\times15 \text{ min.})}{100 \text{ blood draws}} = \frac{450 \text{ min.}}{100 \text{ blood draws}} = 4.5 \text{ min./blood draw}$$

One patient must leave the department every 4.5 minutes or every 270 seconds. In order for this to happen, no single process step can take more than 270 seconds. Think in terms of an assembly line where a product, perhaps an automobile, comes off the assembly line every fifteen minutes. Obviously it takes longer than fifteen minutes to build a car, but every fifteen minutes the assembly line advances and the car at the last process step is completed. In similar fashion, each patient in the process must advance to the next process step every 270 seconds.

To start the map, begin by drawing the three processes and their related information (see Figure 4.4).

The fact that patients are waiting between each process step indicates that inventory exists in the form of excess patients. Inventory is always an indicator that patients are being pushed between processes. Patients are processed on a first-come, first-served basis; also known as first-in first-out or FIFO. Patients waiting at each process step are represented by an inventory triangle including numbers that indicate the minimum and maximum inventory levels. Push arrows used to connect the processes indicate that patients are being pushed from one process to the next. Sequencing is defined as first-in, first-out at each process (see Figure 4.5).

Because the flow of information is just as important as the physical flow of patients, information flow must now be added to the map. Having patients where they need to be when they need to be there but without the information necessary to provide service is non-value-added.

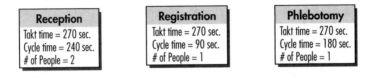

FIGURE 4.4   Process boxes displaying process-related information.

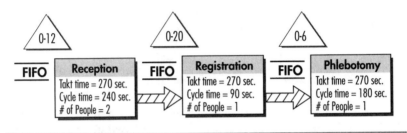

FIGURE 4.5   Example of flow, sequencing, and inventory in the value stream.

Information flow begins when the physician's office faxes a test request to the Laboratory. Orders are entered into the database, where they may be easily accessed by the registrar during the registration process. Patient demographic information is uploaded to the database during the registration process. This initiates the printing of specimen labels in the phlebotomy area (see Figure 4.6). Information boxes are added to the arrows to describe what is being transmitted. When electronic transmission is relayed by means other than data entry to a database, the method should be identified adjacent to the information arrow (that is, phone, fax, and so on).

The final step in the process involves transporting the specimens to the Laboratory for processing at the end of each day. Test results are faxed to the doctor's offices (see Figure 4.7) and the mapping of the entire value stream is now complete. The map includes both the physical flow of the patient and the flow of information and represents the entire process from the receipt of doctors' orders through the delivery of test results. At this point, additional valuable information must be added before moving on to the future state map.

A time line should be drawn at the bottom of the map to indicate the beginning and end of each process (see Figure 4.8). The actual cycle time for each process step is written on the time line below the corresponding process box. Wait times are denoted on the time line between process boxes. The sum of all process times equals the time required to provide the service, the added-value time. The term *value added* is used loosely here to indicate that

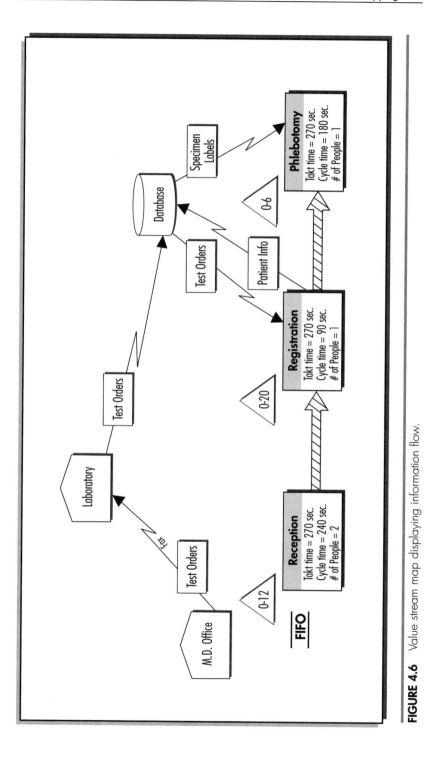

FIGURE 4.6 Value stream map displaying information flow.

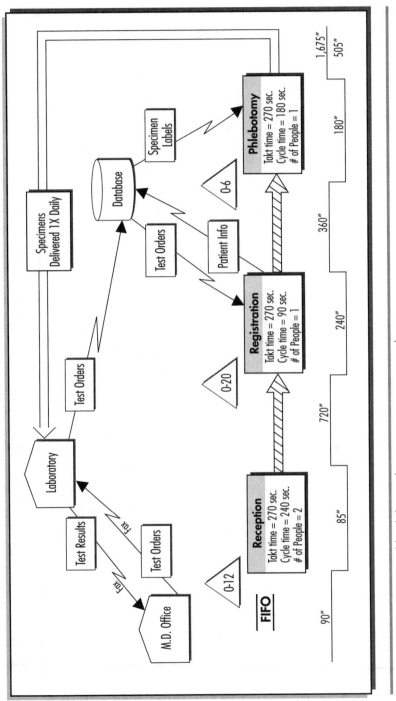

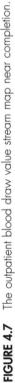

FIGURE 4.7 The outpatient blood draw value stream map near completion.

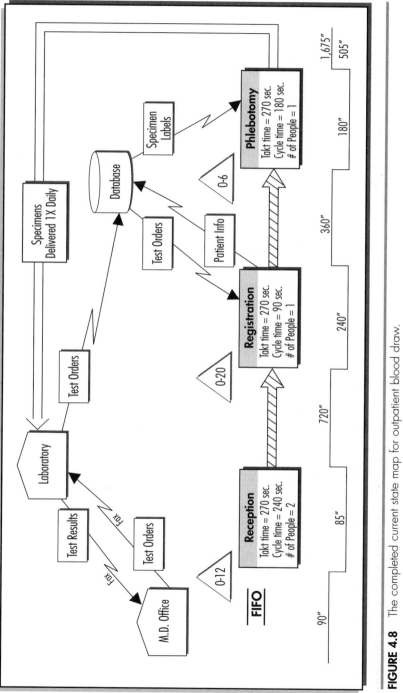

FIGURE 4.8 The completed current state map for outpatient blood draw.

something is happening; the patient is not merely waiting to be processed through the value stream.

By adding all of the values on the time line we calculate lead time. *Lead time* is the time it takes to process one patient through the entire value stream from beginning to end. Like cycle time, lead time is dependent on identifying the customer. From the physician's standpoint, it is the time elapsed between writing the order and receiving the test results. For the patient (represented by this VSM), it may be the entire time spent in the facility. Lead time and value-added time are used to calculate the efficiency of the process, that is, how much of the process is value-added vs. non-value-added. The Process Efficiency Percentage (PEP) is determined by dividing the value-added time by the lead time and multiplying by 100. For this example, the value-added time and lead time are calculated to be 505 minutes and 1,675 minutes, respectively. The process cycle efficiency for the outpatient blood draw process is then calculated as follows:

$$\text{PEP} = \frac{\text{Value-Added Time}}{\text{Lead Time}} = \frac{505 \text{ min.}}{1,675 \text{ min.}} = .301 \text{ or } 30.1\%$$

To complete the map, label it current state, name the process, and include the date the map was drawn (see Figure 4.8). This will avoid confusion later on, when multiple maps exist for the value stream. It will ensure that the most recent map is being referenced.

DRAWING THE FUTURE STATE MAP

The future state map depicts the ideal value stream, the goal of a lean transformation. The future state map should represent the elimination of non-value-added steps, the implementation of a pull system, and the unobstructed flow of the patient or product through the system. The future state map for the University Hospital outpatient blood draw process is shown in Figure 4.9.

Notice that this map no longer includes triangles between the process boxes. This illustrates that patients are now being pulled through the process. With a pull system, there is no patient inventory and, as a result, no waiting. Patient wait time has been reduced to zero. Also note that the information flow has not changed. Since there were no issues with the flow of information, this portion of the map remains the same. The improved turnaround time was achieved by delivering specimens to the lab for processing four times a day, instead of only once at the end of the day. The resulting process efficiency is 100 percent. Remember that this is merely a representation of the ideal future state. In order to achieve this, it is necessary to develop an action plan.

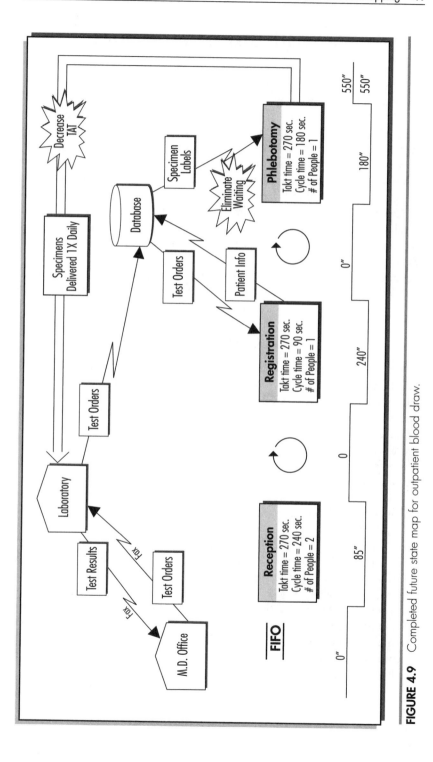

FIGURE 4.9   Completed future state map for outpatient blood draw.

THE VALUE STREAM WORK PLAN

Bear in mind that value stream mapping is only a tool. The current state map depicts where the process is right now, a snapshot in time. It identifies areas to be targeted for improvement.

The future state map illustrates the ideal for each process, a goal to be reached. The benefits of this map will only be realized by achieving the future state. To achieve the future state, a series of lean improvement events must be implemented. These are associated with the improvement explosions icons signifying the action necessary to arrive at the ideal state. It is imperative that these events be scheduled as part of the mapping process. Do not put this off. A lean transformation requires a bias for getting things done. The creation of a value stream work plan is necessary to ensure that the future state will come to fruition. It is project management. The work plan lists the steps necessary to achieve the goal, designates responsibility, specifies the time frame for completion, and provides a visual indicator of progress. A Gantt chart is an excellent tool for creating a value stream work plan. An example of a value stream work plan, created using Microsoft® Project, is illustrated in Figure 4.10.

CONCLUSION

Value stream mapping is a powerful tool, but it is only a tool; by itself, it will not transform the organization. A value stream map is analogous to a set of blueprints for a house. The builder may know what the house is meant to look like—the layout, room sizes, placement of cabinets, fixtures, doors, and windows. A schedule for completion may have been developed with the future owners to be sure that each stage of construction is completed on time in order to ensure completion by a predetermined date. However, without tools and the knowledge of how to use those tools, the house won't be built. It will only be a vision, something that would be nice to have. The same is true for the value stream map. Without the tools and the knowledge of how to implement these tools, the future state will only be something that would be nice to have.

This book provides detailed information on many of the tools necessary for a lean transformation. The knowledge to implement these tools can only be acquired by way of experience. This is where the assistance of a consultant becomes invaluable. A good consultant will work with the designated lean leaders within the organization to transfer knowledge and guide them as they gain experience with these tools. Just as a carpenter's apprentice learns from the master carpenter, lean leaders will learn from the consultant and will eventually be able to work on their own. Be sure to seek a consultant with healthcare/hospital experience.

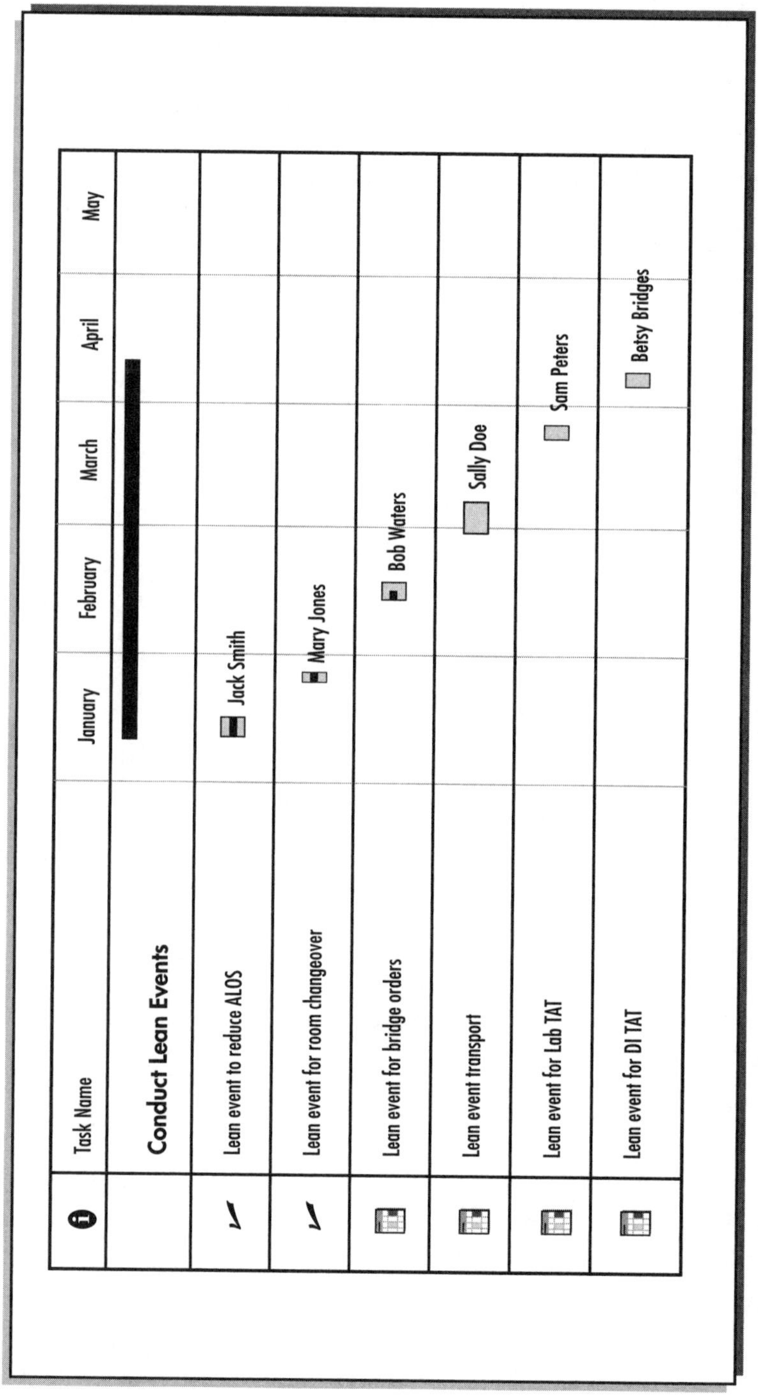

🛈	Task Name	January	February	March	April	May
	Conduct Lean Events	▮▮▮▮▮▮▮▮▮				
↘	Lean event to reduce ALOS	▣ Jack Smith				
↘	Lean event for room changeover	▣▣ Mary Jones				
🗓	Lean event for bridge orders		▣▣ Bob Waters			
🗓	Lean event transport			▣ Sally Doe		
🗓	Lean event for Lab TAT			▣ Sam Peters		
🗓	Lean event for DI TAT				▣ Betsy Bridges	

FIGURE 4.10   Example of a value stream work plan using Microsoft Project.

With the current- and future-state value stream maps in hand, the next step on the lean road map is to develop standard work. The next chapter details the five steps to developing standard work. Some or all of the other tools defined in this book will be utilized during the "Modify the Existing Process" phase of standard work. Since every lean event is unique and since these tools are employed based on the problems associated with each event, subsequent chapters do not represent any structured order for implementation. Use these tools on an as-needed basis.

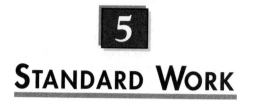

STANDARD WORK

When people are asked to choose the most difficult aspect of any improvement initiative, the one answer that comes back most often is "maintaining the gains." Preventing backsliding is, by far, the most difficult and elusive phase of any improvement project; it is sometimes completely overlooked. Most projects consume a great deal of time—planning, gathering data, brainstorming ideas, implementing change, and verifying results. The improvement team quantifies the results and celebrates their success, only to discover three, six, or twelve months later that everything has gone back to the way it was. The bottom-line benefits of the project are never realized by the organization and the team members wonder why they even bothered.

People will tolerate change, but remembering what "feels right" will often result in doing what they are accustomed to. For this reason, standard work must be integral to any improvement project. Standard work is all about maintaining the gains. Without standard work, there is no continuous improvement. Every member of an organization undergoing a lean transformation must understand and internalize this concept.

In addition to maintaining the gains, standard work incorporates the tools needed to generate change. While value stream mapping looks at the process from thirty thousand feet, standard work uses a magnifying glass, breaking down the process into component tasks that can then be analyzed and improved. Implementing standard work involves five steps, all of which will be addressed in this chapter:

1. Evaluate the current situation

2. Identify areas of opportunity

3. Modify the existing process

4. Substantiate and enumerate improvements

5. Implement new standard work (see Figure 5.1)

Standard work and work standards are often confused. Work standards describe the specific standards relative to the work being done. Standard work describes the sequence of activities necessary to accomplish that work, specifies the time required to complete each task, and verifies that the work is being performed in accordance with patient/customer demand. Standard work is defined as the most effective combination of activities that will minimize non-value-added activities while providing high quality care.

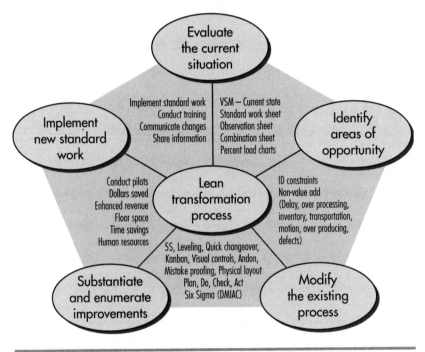

FIGURE 5.1 The five-step method for implementing standard work.

DEFINITIONS

Before proceeding with the implementation of standard work, it is important to know the definition of these terms and understand how they apply to Lean: work sequence, standard work in process, and curtain.

WORK SEQUENCE

This is the sequence in which activities are performed by one person to complete one cycle time. Work sequence and process sequence are not necessarily the same thing. The process sequence could be the sequence of tasks performed by one or more people to complete one process cycle time. For example, the process sequence for a nuclear stress test includes a work sequence for the Cardio Tech, the Nuclear Tech, and the Cardiologist. Each has his or her own work sequence; together they make up the process sequence.

SWIP

SWIP is an acronym for Standard Work In Process. This is the minimum number of patients or products required to ensure flow by maintaining the process sequence. In a pull system, the target for SWIP is always one patient or product. To accomplish this, it is necessary to balance the operation cycle times among staff members so as to meet takt time. In so doing, a pull system is maintained and SWIP is kept at a level of one. To better understand SWIP, imagine three separate operations within a process (see Figure 5.2). The takt time for the process is 310 seconds. The cycle times for operations 1, 2 and 3 are 250 seconds, 300 seconds, and 300 seconds, respectively. Since all three cycle times are less than takt time we know that we can meet customer demand. Notice, however, that the cycle time for operation 1 is 50 seconds less than operations 2 and 3. This means that inventory will build up between operations 1 and 2. In lean terms, operation 1 will be pushing patients to operation 2, rather than operation 2 pulling patients from operation 1. To achieve a SWIP of one patient, operation 1 should not release the current patient until operation 2 is complete and ready to pull a patient from the upstream process. This means that the person performing operation 1 must wait until the person performing operation 2 has completed an operation cycle. Ideally, this waiting time is utilized performing some value-added function and not by actually waiting. Another option would be to balance the operation cycle times by shifting work from operations 2 and 3 to operation 1. The tool used to determine the feasibility of this option is called a Percent Load Chart, discussed later in this chapter.

When a process has one product or patient at each operation and one product or patient as SWIP, we refer to this as having the line loaded.

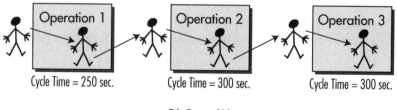

Operation 1	Operation 2	Operation 3
Cycle Time = 250 sec.	Cycle Time = 300 sec.	Cycle Time = 300 sec.

Takt Time = 310 sec.

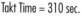

FIGURE 5.2 Example of one-piece flow demonstrating SWIP.

In manufacturing, a production line can end the day loaded. When the workers return the next day, they begin working with a loaded line. Process flow commences with the very first product off the line. This is often not possible in healthcare. Here the line must be loaded each day before flow can be attained.

CURTAIN

There are some instances when it is not possible to maintain SWIP at one. In these cases, a tool called a curtain is implemented, allowing SWIP to be maintained at a level necessary to sustain flow.

Consider a process that requires an incubation period for specimens. The operations to be performed before and after incubation may require very short cycle times, but incubation may take 10 minutes. For demonstrative purposes we assign a cycle time of 30 seconds to the operations that precede and follow incubation. In order to maintain a SWIP of one, it would be necessary to wait 10 minutes during the processing of each specimen and a specimen would be completed every 10 minutes and 30 seconds at best. Using a curtain permits the processing of one specimen every 30 seconds once the line is loaded, thereby maintaining flow.

To set up a curtain, first balance all preceding and subsequent operations as closely as possible. Next, divide the incubation time by the longest of the remaining cycle times. In this example, the result is twenty (10 minutes/ 30 seconds). This is the value of SWIP to use in the curtain. To load the line, conduct the preceding operations until twenty specimens are loaded into the incubator. While these twenty specimens are incubating, prepare the next twenty specimens. When the first incubation period is complete, remove the twenty specimens from the incubator and load the next twenty. The line is now loaded and the curtain is established. From this point on, flow may be maintained at a rate of one specimen every 30 seconds. The process steps proceed as follows:

1. Prepare a specimen for incubation

2. Finish processing one of the twenty specimens previously removed from the incubator

3. Repeat the first two steps until twenty specimens have been processed

4. Unload the incubator and reload with the prepared specimens

5. Repeat from step one

The only interruption to flow is the time necessary to load and unload the incubator.

STEP 1. EVALUATING THE CURRENT SITUATION

Evaluating the current situation, the first step in the five-step process for implementing standard work, is accomplished using the four standard work forms. Any organization undergoing a lean transformation must be intimately familiar with the standard work sheet, the time observation sheet, the combination sheet, and the percent load chart. Each of these forms will be covered in detail in this section.

STANDARD WORK SHEET

The first step to implementing standard work is to document the existing work sequence. This is accomplished by tracking, on paper, the path of the person or people performing the process tasks. The form used for this phase is called a standard work sheet (see Figure 5.3). The standard work sheet is often referred to as a spaghetti diagram or spaghetti chart because the lines drawn to trace the operation sequence often resemble a plate of spaghetti.

To create a standard work sheet, begin by drawing rectangles or squares on the sheet to represent the different areas accessed as part of the process. In essence, you are creating a simplified floor plan of the work area. Next choose a starting point, write the number one at that point, and circle it. Then place the pencil on the paper at the starting point and trace the route the person takes in performing the next process step.

At that point, write the number 2 and circle it, trace the route to the next process step, and so on. If the person has completed one work or process sequence and is beginning the next, draw a dotted line to connect the last step to the first step. Do this for all the people performing the process. To differentiate between the different people, use a different colors for each. The symbol for a person performing a process is shown in Figure 5.4. Draw one symbol for each person involved in the process steps. If a quality check is required at any point (for example, checking for drug interactions and compatibility), draw a diamond shape at that step. Draw the cross symbol if a safety precaution, such as using a needle box, is part of the process step. If inventory accumulates at any process step, draw a triangle to indicate SWIP inventory and indicate the level or range inside or below the triangle.

Also included on the standard work sheet is a box for cycle time and takt time. The cycle time required here is the process cycle time, the sum of all the operation cycle times if one person is performing the process. If more than one person is performing the process, the process cycle time will be the greater of the sums of the work sequence cycle times.

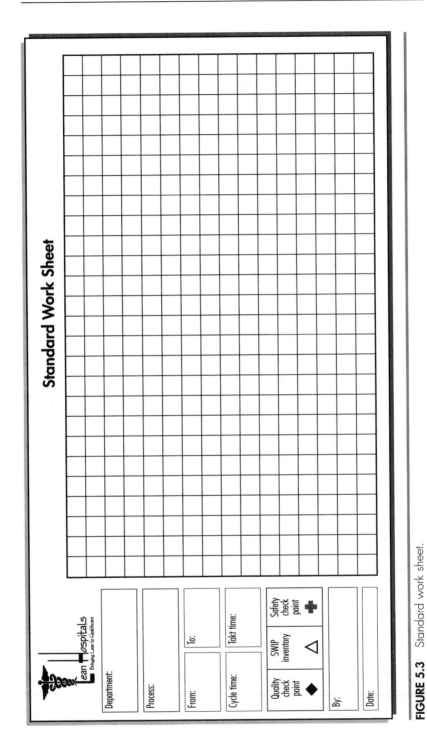

FIGURE 5.3　Standard work sheet.

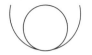

FIGURE 5.4 Symbol for a person performing a process.

The completed sheet provides information relative to the current situation regarding excess motion and transport in a process. Minimizing these non-value-added activities in as many operations as possible creates flow. This can be accomplished by rearranging the work area to compliment the process flow. Ideally, the operations should be arranged in sequence so that the cycle ends close to where it begins again.

Figure 5.5 is an example of a u-shaped cell employing two people. Notice that the work sequence for each operator differs from the process sequence. The entire process goes from operation 1 to operation 6, while the work sequence for operator one is 1, 2, 3 and for operator two is 4, 5, 6. In this example the cycle time is less than the takt time, which means the process meets customer demand. If customer demand increased, takt time would go down and more people would be needed for the process. Alternatively, reducing operation cycle times would also meet takt time. If takt time increased, demand could be met with fewer people.

In order to obtain accurate information relative to cycle time, it is necessary to break the process down into individual operations and actually determine how much time is required to complete each step. To accomplish this, the Time Observation Sheet is employed

TIME OBSERVATION SHEET

The next form used to implement standard work is the time observation sheet (see Figure 5.6). The purpose of this form is to document the time required to complete the specific operations that make up the process (cycle time) and to identify the non-value-added steps in the process. Time observations are done to determine where and how the process breaks down. For example, if a person completes five cycles under takt time and the sixth cycle takes significantly longer, the reason for that longer cycle time must be determined and action taken to correct the anomaly. This should be done in order to ensure that takt time is met every time the process is performed.

It is important to conduct time observations in order to accurately evaluate the current situation. Written procedures or other documentation only provide information as to how the process is meant to be performed, not what actually happens. This point is critical to the successful implementation of the improvement initiative. It is also imperative that anyone conducting time observations focus on the person performing the tasks, not on the product or

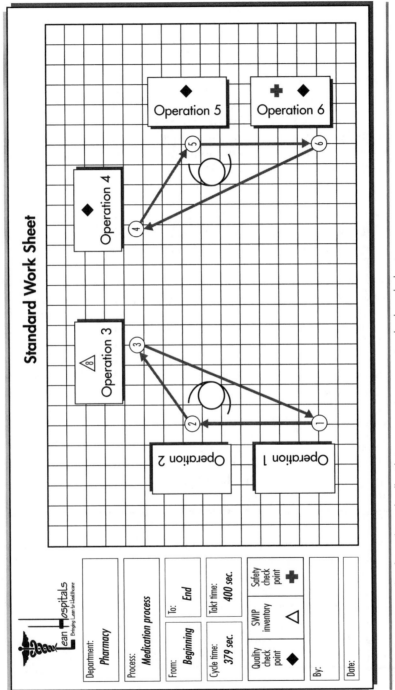

FIGURE 5.5 Example of a u-shaped cell with two operators on a standard work sheet.

Lean Hospitals
Bringing Lean to Healthcare

Time Observation Sheet

Process observed:

Observer:

Date:

Task	Task Description	1	2	3	4	5	6	7	8	9	10	Best Time	Remarks
1													
2													
3													
4													
5													
6													
7													
8													
9													
10													
11													
12													
13													
14													
15													
Observed cycle time:													

FIGURE 5.6 Time observation sheet.

service and not on the equipment. The time observation form and a stop watch or other timing device are essential tools for timing the individual operations.

When conducting time observations, first observe the sequence in which the work is performed. Do not be concerned, at this point, with how long it takes to perform the sequence. Determine first if there is some repetitiveness to the steps being performed. If the steps taken by the individual performing the operation(s) or process are completely random, determine a sequence and instruct the individual to follow the specified routine for the purpose of time observations. Once a sequence is established, the next step is to define the individual tasks required to complete the operation(s) or process. The focus here is on the work sequence rather than process sequence. This means that a separate time observation sheet is required for each person in the process. If more than one person is performing the process sequence, complete a separate time observation form for each person. Always complete a separate time observation sheet for each person.

Once defined, enter the individual tasks on the time observation form in the "Task Description" column. The person performing the work sequence will begin the process on a signal from the observer that timing has begun. If using a stop watch, allow the watch to run until all the desired observations are completed. Stopping and restarting after each task results in editing the actual time required to perform the task. As the process goes on, write the time at which each operation is completed in the un-shaded box (top half) corresponding to the task description in the first observation column. When the process is complete, move to the next observation column and record the time in the un-shaded box for each task. Continue recording until a sufficient number of observations have been recorded. The "rule of thumb" regarding time observations: the more, the better. Be sure to include both value-added and non-value-added times, but do not combine them as a single task. For example, if a technician must walk over to a work station, obtain an item, and return to the original position, define this as three different tasks—walk, get item, and return. Describing the task as "get item" does not highlight the non-value-added walking segment.

The observed times are written in the appropriate box for each set of observations as they happen, not as they are supposed to happen. If there is an interruption, timing continues. The actual time is entered in the appropriate box, and a note is added to the "remarks" column. This remarks column is important to the observation study. In fact, it may be the the the most important column on the form. It highlights reasons for variation in the process sequence such as interruptions, unusual occurrences, and non-value-added activities such as searching or waiting. As a result, it illuminates opportunities for improvement. When adding a note to the remarks column, indicate to which observation the remark is associated (for example, "observation 4, nurse answered the phone").

Ask questions for clarification after observing, not before or while you are observing. If you ask a question while observing, the person being observed may stop what they are doing to answer. This will disrupt the sequence and provide erroneous times. Instead, make a note of the question and ask it later.

Observe times for at least five cycles. The more cycles observed, the more opportunity to expose non-value-added occurrences. When sufficient observations have been completed, use a red pen to record the time of the first observation in the shaded box associated with the first task. To fill the remaining shaded boxes, subtract the recorded time for the previous operation from the time recorded for the current operation. Enter this value in the corresponding shaded box. Continue to do this until an operation task time is calculated for all observations. Record task times in the shaded boxes using a red pen. This makes it easier to differentiate between recorded time and task time.

In the column labeled "Best Time," record the lowest task time observed for the related task. To complete the form, tally up the times from each observation column and the "Best Time" column and enter the number in the "Observed Cycle Time" boxes on the bottom of the form. An example of a completed Time observation form is shown in Figure 5.7. The "Best Time" column is the official cycle time for this process as it currently exists.

During the fourth observation of the removal of the blood pressure cuff, the nurse noticed that the dial on the blood pressure cuff was broken. After a brief search, the spare cuff was located and the cycle resumed. This anomaly caused an interruption in the cycle; immediate action is required to replace the defective cuff. If action is not taken, the next nurse who has a problem with a blood pressure cuff will discover that the spare is also defective, resulting in a more substantial delay.

A useful tool for time observations is a video camera. Video taping the process allows observation without interrupting the process flow. The video camera can be set up on a tripod in an out-of-the-way area and left there to record the process. Check with the Human Resources department before setting up and using any video taping equipment. The hospital may have a policy about taking pictures or videos of employees and may require written permission from employees in the area being recorded. If video taping is permitted, be sure to inform people why they are being filmed. They may feel uncomfortable at first, but it won't be long before they are back in the rhythm and performing their duties normally. Video taping also offers the opportunity to rewind and observe things that might have been missed as a result of an interruption or other distraction. If questions arise, the video can be stopped and explanations given without affecting flow. Lastly, if observations need to be done on off shifts, the camera can be set up and programmed to start recording at a time later in the day.

Time
Observation
Sheet

Lean Hospitals
Bringing Lean to Healthcare

Process observed:
Observe vital signs

Observer:
John Doe

Date:
01-01-2001

Task	Task Description	1	2	3	4	5	6	7	8	9	10	Best Time	Remarks
1	Time pulse and record	:58 / 58	4:08 / 43	7:31 / 53	10:57 / 57							43	
2	Get thermometer	1:06 / 8	4:17 / 9	7:40 / 9	11:05 / 8							8	
3	Take temperature and record	2:11 / 65	5:26 / 69	8:46 / 66	12:01 / 66							65	
4	Return thermometer	2:18 / 7	5:34 / 8	8:46 / 10	12:08 / 7							7	
5	Get blood pressure cuff	2:31 / 13	5:49 / 15	9:00 / 14	13:29 / 81							13	Observation 4 cuff is broken, nurse cannot find spare
6	Obtain blood pressure and record	3:13 / 42	6:27 / 38	9:39 / 39	14:06 / 37							37	
7	Return blood pressure cuff	3:25 / 12	6:38 / 11	9:50 / 11	14:18 / 12							11	
8													
9													
10													
11													
12													
13													
14													
15													
	Observed cycle time:	3:25	3:13	3:22	4:28							3:04	

FIGURE 5.7   Example of a time observation sheet with observations for vital signs.

Be sure to use the date/time feature available on almost all cameras when video taping. Using this feature eliminates the need for a separate timing device.

COMBINATION SHEET

The next step in the implementation of standard work is to complete a combination sheet. The combination sheet, as the name implies, is used to record manual, walking, automatic, and waiting times in a single graphical, easy-to-read representation of a process. It identifies excess capacity and non-value-added process steps and assists in the development of a more efficient combination of these different characteristics of the process. A blank combination sheet is shown in Figure 5.8.

Begin by adding a scale across the top of the graph that will allow representation of the process. Draw solid lines to represent manual operations. Use dotted lines for automatic time and wavy lines for walking time. Use a double line to represent time spent waiting between the end of the cycle and takt time. When the last operation is drawn, the line is returned to the top of the graph indicating the start of the next cycle. A red line drawn down the page signifies takt time.

Transfer to the combination sheet the information acquired on the time observation sheet relative to the tasks and their cycle times. Note that walking is not an operation. It is how the person being observed transitions from one task to the next. Using our time observation sheet example for obtaining vital signs (Figure 5.7), we see that there are only three operations: time pulse and record, take temperature and record, and obtain blood pressure and record. The other times observed should be entered in the walk column and represented on the graph accordingly, using a wavy line. Since taking temperature involves placing a thermometer in the patient's mouth and waiting sixty seconds, it is represented on the graph as automatic time using a dotted line. Automatic time is interpreted as waiting time unless the person being observed is performing another task while waiting. An example of a completed combination sheet for "obtaining vital signs" is shown in Figure 5.9. It becomes immediately obvious that by eliminating the walking associated with this process, the cycle time can be reduced by 39 seconds. By simply moving the thermometer and blood pressure cuff to the point of use, walking is eliminated and the process can be completed within the takt time.

Waiting time always provides an opportunity for improvement. With sixty seconds of waiting time in this process, the improvement team has two options. They may suggest that the nurse take the patient's blood pressure while waiting for the oral thermometer reading, or use a digital ear thermometer to obtain the patient's temperature. Figure 5.10 shows a combination sheet for the process after the oral thermometer was replaced with a digital ear thermometer. The time required for this task has been reduced to five seconds, and all walking time

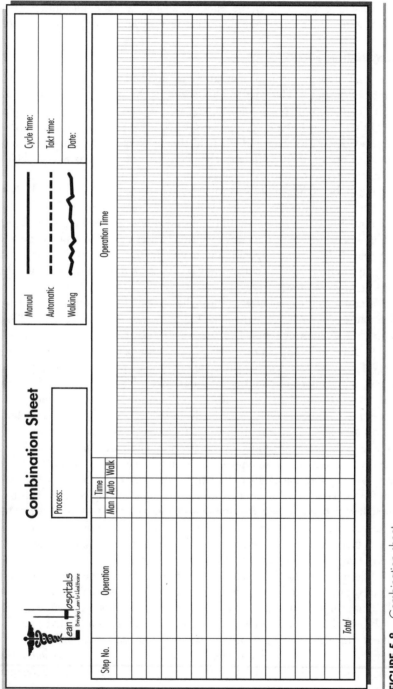

FIGURE 5.8 Combination sheet.

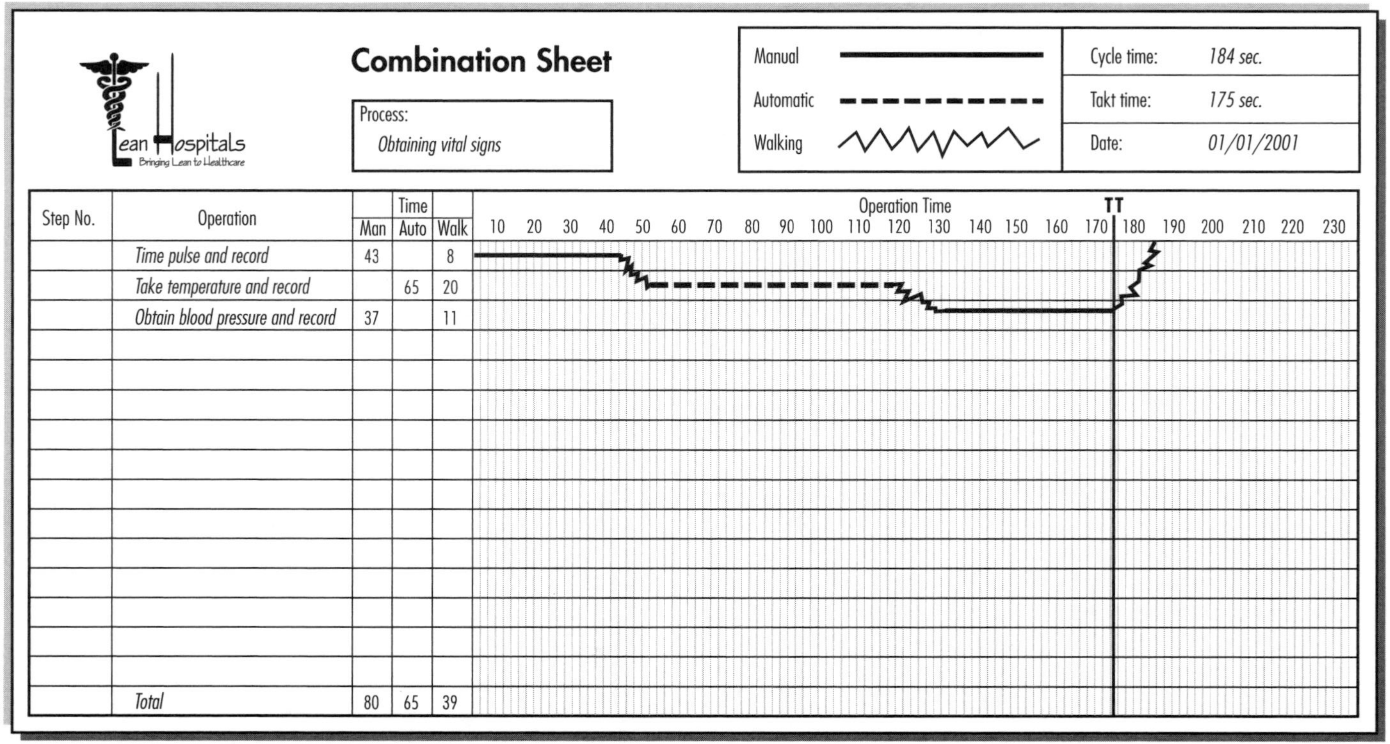
Lean Hospitals
Bringing Lean to Healthcare
Combination Sheet
Process:
Obtaining vital signs
Manual
Automatic
Walking
Cycle time: 184 sec.
Takt time: 175 sec.
Date: 01/01/2001
Step No.
Operation
Time
Man
Auto
Walk
Time pulse and record
43
8
Take temperature and record
65
20
Obtain blood pressure and record
37
11
Total
80
65
39
Operation Time
TT
10 20 30 40 50 60 70 80 90 100 110 120 130 140 150 160 170 180 190 200 210 220 230

FIGURE 5.9 Completed combination sheet for vital signs before improvements.

has been eliminated. A double line between the end of the cycle and the red takt time line indicates available process time.

This is a simple example devised for illustrative purposes, but the method works for all processes. Because the cycle time is less than the takt time, the process easily meets customer demand. In fact, the cycle time has been reduced so significantly that the nurse can process two patients within the takt time. If two nurses were being utilized to perform vital signs, the second nurse is now free to take on other duties related to patient care.

PERCENT LOAD CHART

The fourth form associated with standard work is the percent load chart. This form is basically a piece of graph paper on which bars are drawn to indicate the cycle time for each person in a process. The x axis represents the individuals performing the tasks and the y axis represents the time required for each individual to complete their cycle. The percent load chart is a useful tool for determining if the work load is well balanced and what staffing levels are required to meet takt time. The percent load chart in Figure 5.11 indicates a workload not evenly distributed and a process that will not meet customer demand. Redistributing the work load, if possible, will allow the process to meet takt time. If these operations include non-value-added steps such as walking, excess motion, waiting, and transportation, eliminating these actions may be enough to bring the operation times below takt time. Another option would be to redefine the process sequence so that the work can be accomplished by four techs instead of five. The additional tech could then be assigned to other value-added processes.

By dividing the manual time required for all the operations in the process by the takt time, it's possible to calculate the number of people required to perform the operation. The process illustrated in Figure 5.11 requires five techs based on demand, as illustrated in the calculation below.

$$\frac{60 + 110 + 105 + 135 + 75}{100} \quad = \quad \frac{485}{100} \quad = \quad 4.85 \text{ Techs} = 5 \text{ Techs}$$

If the first operation in this process required 100 seconds instead of 60 seconds, the total process time would equal 525 seconds; six techs would be required to meet demand.

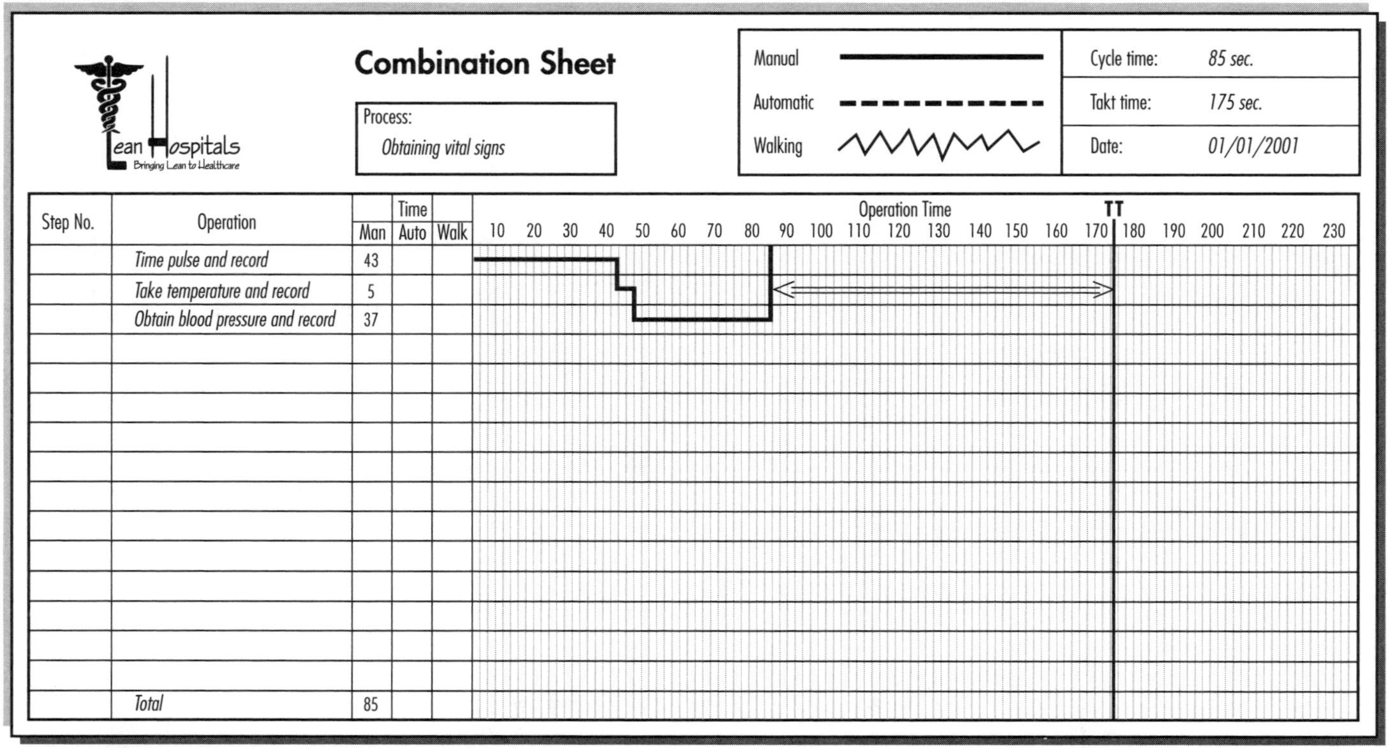
Lean Hospitals
Bringing Lean to Healthcare
Combination Sheet
Process:
Obtaining vital signs
Manual
Automatic
Walking
Cycle time: 85 sec.
Takt time: 175 sec.
Date: 01/01/2001
Step No.
Operation
Time
Man
Auto
Walk
Time pulse and record
43
Take temperature and record
5
Obtain blood pressure and record
37
Total
85
Operation Time
TT
10 20 30 40 50 60 70 80 90 100 110 120 130 140 150 160 170 180 190 200 210 220 230

FIGURE 5.10 Completed combination sheet for vital signs after improvements.

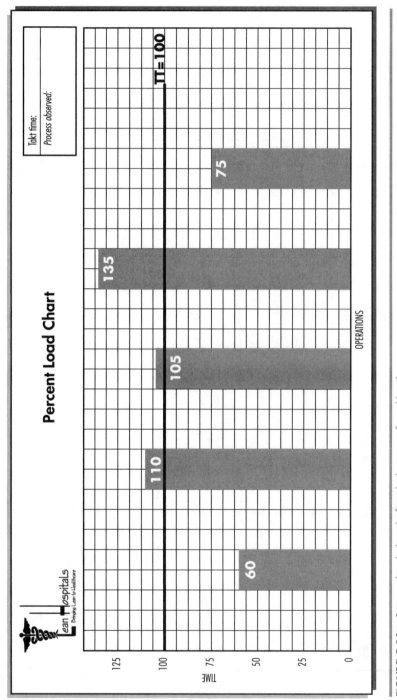

FIGURE 5.11 Percent load chart before balancing of workload.

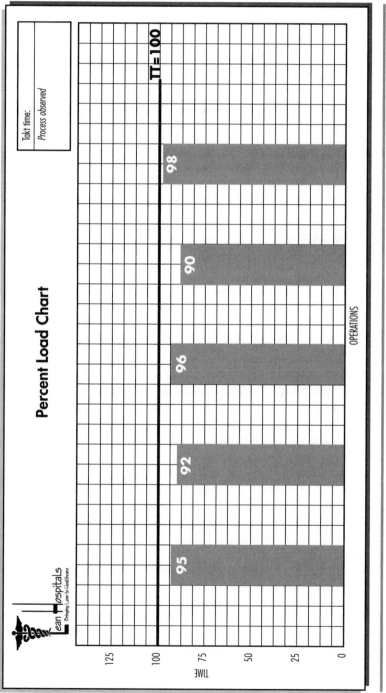

FIGURE 5.12   Percent load chart after balancing of workload.

Notice, however, that although there are enough techs to meet demand, the process will fail to meet the goal of one part or patient every 100 seconds because three of the processes take longer than takt time. To correct this, it is necessary to eliminate any non-value-added steps and/or redistribute the workload as shown in Figure 5.12.

STEP 2. IDENTIFYING AREAS OF OPPORTUNITY

The second step for implementing standard work is to identify areas of opportunity. These are areas where flow is interrupted, where inventories of patients or products accumulate, or where the system breaks down. Non-value-added steps must be identified as such and later eliminated. Seven areas have been identified where non-value-added operations are prevalent:

1. Delay
2. Over processing
3. Inventory
4. Transportation
5. Motion
6. Over producing
7. Making defects

An organization's pursuit of non-value-added operations should not be restricted to these seven areas. They are meant to provide a starting point in the identification of non-value-added operations and are by no means all-inclusive. These steps, with examples applicable to healthcare, are elaborated on in Table 5.1.

Surprisingly, the identification of these seven areas of non-value-added activity is a difficult task. A key point here is that being busy is not necessarily adding value. People performing a process may be busy 110% of the time and yet not add value. Repeatedly calling the Laboratory to obtain test results, making a trip to the storeroom to find an urgently needed item, or attending to fifteen pre-op patients when there are only four operating rooms all involve work. They do not necessarily add value. The success of any lean initiative is dependent on the team's ability to discern the value-added and non-value-added components of a process. Value stream maps and standard work forms assist lean teams by making non-value-added steps obvious. Team members, however, must possess the ability to identify these steps and be willing to acknowledge that they are, indeed, non-value-added. Acknowledging that a process step is non-value-added is, by far, the most difficult aspect of identifying opportunities for improvement. The individuals performing the process steps will devise a myriad of reasons why each operation must be performed the way they are performing it, and take a firm stand against

TABLE 5.1   The seven wastes identified by Taiichi Ohno and examples from healthcare.

Delay	Waiting for bed assignments, waiting to be discharged, waiting for treatment, waiting for diagnostic tests, waiting for supplies, waiting for approval, waiting for the doctor, waiting for the nurse
Over processing	Excessive paperwork, redundant processes, unnecessary tests, using an IV when oral medication would suffice, multiple bed moves, requiring approval for "sure things"
Inventory	Lab specimens awaiting analysis, ED patients awaiting a bed assignment, patients awaiting diagnostic tests, excess supplies kept on hand just in case, dictation awaiting transcription
Transportation	Transporting lab specimens, transporting patients, transporting medication, transporting supplies
Motion	Searching for charts and supplies, delivering meds, nurses caring for patients on different wings
Over production	Mixing drugs in anticipation of patient needs, forcing admit to ICU or monitored bed when not necessary
Defects	Medication errors, wrong-site surgery, improper labeling of specimens, multiple sticks for blood draws, injury caused by defect drugs or restraints or lack of restraints, failing to administer antibiotics on time

modifying it in any way. Occasionally these reasons are rooted in reality and the non-value-added component must be performed as it always has been. Most of the time these steps can be modified or even eliminated without consequence. It is important for employees to know that their personal effort is not "non-value-added." It's the task that needs reform.

One way to identify non-value-added process steps is to complete a Value Process Chart. All tasks performed as part of a process can be categorized as an operation, transportation, delay, storage, or inspection. Each of these tasks is represented by a symbol as indicated on the form in Figure 5.13. Using the tasks identified on the time observation sheet for "obtaining vital signs" (see Figure 5.7), chart the process by drawing a line connecting the category that relates to the description. Include the distance traveled, the quantity, and the time taken to perform each step, as applicable. Summarize the number of tasks associated with each category and the time required to accomplish all tasks in each category. Note the distance traveled. In the "possibilities" column, identify the opportunities/approach to improving the process. Chart the proposed process and summarize the information for the new process and calculate the differences relative to each category.

Value Process Chart

Lean Hospitals
Bringing Lean to Healthcare

Summary

	Present		Proposed		Diff.	
	No.	Time	No.	Time	No.	Time
○ Operation	3	140	3	97		
⇨ Transport	4	39	0	0		
□ Delay						
◇ Store						
△ Inspect						
Dst Traveled	ft.		ft.		ft.	

Date:	*01-01-2001*
Process:	*Obtaining vital signs*
Chart begins:	*Pulse*
Chart ends:	*Returning BP cuff*

										POSSIBILITIES						
												CHANGE				
No.	Description of present method	OPERATION	TRANSPORT	DELAY	STORE	INSPECT	DIST. IN FEET	QUANTITY	TIME	ELIMINATE	COMBINE	SEQUENCE	PLACE	PERSON	IMPROVE	Notes
1	*Time pulse and record*	○	⇨	□	◇	△			43	x	x					
2	*Get thermometer*	○	⇨	□	◇	△	5		8	x						*Move thermometer to POU*
3	*Take temperature and record*	○	⇨	□	◇	△			60		x	x				*Start temp before pulse*
4	*Return thermometer*	○	⇨	□	◇	△	5		7	x						
5	*Get BP cuff*	○	⇨	□	◇	△	10		13	x						*Move blood pressure cuff to POU*
6	*Obtain BP and record*	○	⇨	□	◇	△			37							
7	*Return BP cuff*	○	⇨	□	◇	△	10		11	x						
8		○	⇨	□	◇	△										
9		○	⇨	□	◇	△										
10		○	⇨	□	◇	△										
11		○	⇨	□	◇	△										
12		○	⇨	□	◇	△										
13		○	⇨	□	◇	△										
14		○	⇨	□	◇	△										
15		○	⇨	□	◇	△										
16		○	⇨	□	◇	△										
17		○	⇨	□	◇	△										
18		○	⇨	□	◇	△										
19		○	⇨	□	◇	△										
20		○	⇨	□	◇	△										
21		○	⇨	□	◇	△										
22		○	⇨	□	◇	△										
23		○	⇨	□	◇	△										
24		○	⇨	□	◇	△										
25		○	⇨	□	◇	△										

FIGURE 5.13 Value process chart.

STEP 3. MODIFYING THE EXISTING PROCESS

Once the current situation has been evaluated and opportunities for improvement identified, ideas must be generated that will modify the existing process in order to realize the benefits. Brainstorming is an excellent method for generating improvement ideas and a good starting point for this step of standard work. Some improvement methods will be obvious and will not require brainstorming. Familiarity with lean concepts makes it easy to recognize how the application of lean tools and/or principles can provide a solution to a problem. Some of the lean concepts used to improve flow, eliminate constraints, and eradicate non-value-added steps include 5S, *Kanban*, *Visual Controls*, *Quick changeover*, *Andon*, *Five Whys*, *Leveling*, and *Mistake Proofing*.

BRAINSTORMING

Although most people are familiar with brainstorming, only a few actually facilitate this process well. Following established guidelines will help you get the most from a brainstorming session. First and most important, never evaluate ideas during the brainstorming session. This will squelch imagination and limit the number of suggestions. Wild ideas should be encouraged, as should building on other people's ideas. Strive for quantity, the more the better. Later in the process, everyone will have the opportunity to analyze the ideas.

There are several approaches to conducting a brainstorming session. The freewheeling method encourages people to call out ideas as they arise. This method, however, may limit participation to the dominant members of the group. The card method is another approach and works well when anonymity is required. Participants simply write ideas on a piece of paper or an index card. The most common approach is the round robin, which allows each person, in turn, to provide an idea. Participants may pass on one turn and provide ideas on subsequent rounds. The facilitator continues to go around the room until everyone runs out of ideas.

If possible, the ideas should be stated in three words or less so the facilitator can jot them on a flip chart and move on to the next idea without losing momentum. It is a good idea to alternate marker colors with each new idea written and to number them as they are written on the flip chart. This will aid in distinguishing between ideas during the next phase of the process.

The next step is list reduction, which involves analyzing the list and reducing it, if necessary, by eliminating duplicate ideas and ideas that may be irrelevant, inappropriate, not feasible, or beyond the control of the group. Never cross out anyone's ideas; just draw a circle or box around them with a red marker. This allows the group to go back to them later in the process, if necessary. At this point, the ideas may be grouped, prioritized, and/or implemented.

ANDON

Andon is derived from the Japanese word for light. It is a visual signal used to indicate an abnormal condition. An andon is sometimes associated with an audio alarm such as a bell or buzzer. The purpose of an andon is to immediately alert the appropriate parties that an abnormal condition exists and requires their immediate attention.

There are four basic styles of andons: the paging andon, the caution andon, the equipment andon, and the normal andon. Each style is usually associated with a color and is standardized throughout the organization. For example, a paging andon may be yellow, caution red, equipment blue, and normal green.

The paging andon is most often associated with a kanban; it is used to signal a request for supplies, forms, or even people. A caution andon signals a condition that will negatively affect the flow of patients or products; it requires immediate intervention on the part of management. A computer problem at registration would generate a caution andon. Equipment andons are used to signal operating status of equipment such as CT scanners, refrigerators, or Gamma cameras. Lastly, the normal andon lamp is lit when things are operating normally.

Usually, three or four andons are associated with a process and provide management with at-a-glance knowledge of the process status.

FIVE WHYS

Another lean concept is known as the Five Whys. The Five Whys are part of a simple technique used to determine the root cause of a problem. This technique involves repeatedly asking *why* until the root cause is identified. On average, this only requires five iterations. The drawback to this concept is that it can be incredibly annoying. It is reminiscent of a four-year-old repeatedly asking *why* to a series of parental responses. For this reason, this concept should be employed carefully. It is highly recommended that structured questions be used in the query such as, "If the tube cannot handle the load, why have we not upgraded to a high performance x-ray tube?" rather than repeatedly saying *Why?* in response to each answer. This is not intended to discourage the use of the Five Whys. On the contrary, because of its simplicity in determining possible root causes, its use should be encouraged. This information is provided simply to caution readers against assaulting their colleagues with a barrage of *whys*. Instead, formulate pointed and specific inquiries.

Implementation of this simple tool is beneficial. It is easy to use, does not require forms or tools, does not involve extensive training and, most importantly, it works. Keep in mind, however, that there may be several root causes to a problem. The Five Whys technique will only lead to one of them at a time. Return to the problem and repeat the process to uncover other causes until the problem is corrected.

LEVELING

Leveling is basically mixed model production. It is a method of sequencing orders for a product or service in a cyclical arrangement in order to provide an even distribution of that product or service. Although flow may seem like a simple concept, actual implementation can often be complicated. The goal of leveling is to create flow based on volume and product mix. Leveling creates a more produce-to-order system.

To provide a simple example, assume a pharmacy receives 100 orders for IV Admixtures each day and works only one shift with one dedicated tech. The takt time would be 4.5 minutes per mixture ($((8x60)-(2x15))/100$). To complicate the issue, however, these mixtures can comprise more than 130 drugs. Luckily, they fall into just three categories: Easy mix, Average mix, and Difficult mix. The cycle times are 2 minutes, 4 minutes, and 8 minutes, respectively. The product mix is 30 Easy mixes, 50 Average mixes, and 20 difficult mixes. By implementing once-a-day production methods, all the Easy mixes would be completed first, the Average mixes next, and the Difficult mixes last. This method, however, does not allow the pharmacy to respond to customer orders.

To create a better production mix and allow the pharmacy the ability to better produce-to-order, leveling is incorporated. The first step is to determine the ratios of each product to the total. For this example the ratios are 30/100 or 3:10 for the Easy mix, 50/100 or 1:2 for the Average mix, and 20/100 or 1:5 for the Difficult mix. For every ten mixes the pharmacy produces, three must be Easy, 5 must be Average, and 2 must be Difficult. If the pharmacy mixes drugs based on the model shown in Figure 5.14, their output will meet customer needs. By implementing this model, the pharmacy produces mixes as shown and then begins again at the beginning of the cycle. Hence, the next four products would be Average-Easy-Average-Difficult and not Average-Difficult-Average-Easy.

The cycle can be run ten times in the 450 minutes available; it will easily meet the requirement for 30 Easy mixes, 50 Average mixes, and 20 Difficult mixes. The system, then, allows the pharmacy to better meet customer needs and takt time. Leveling provides the flexibility to make what the customers want, when they want it, in the quantity they want. It also reduces the risk of overproducing based on past orders and then having to discard the excess.

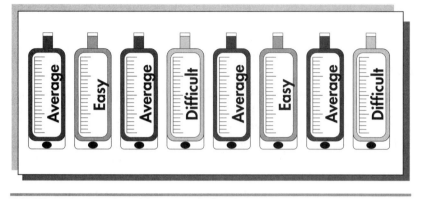

FIGURE 5.14   Mixed modeling example for pharmacy.

STEP 4. SUBSTANTIATING AND ENUMERATING IMPROVEMENTS

Implementing a full-scale process modification that has not been verified, even for a short period of time, can generate disorder within a department. Substantiating the modifications being proposed before full-scale implementation is highly recommended. This is most often accomplished by means of pilot runs that allow glitches to surface on a small scale without affecting normal operations.

Once the improvements have been implemented on a full-scale level, verify that expected results are being realized. Quantify the results in cost reduction, revenue generation, time savings, defects avoided, floor space availability, turnaround time reduction, and so on. Savings that may be "soft" or intangibles should be included also.

STEP 5. IMPLEMENT NEW STANDARD WORK

Developing a new standard that reflects the implemented improvements is the final and most critical step in the implementation of standard work, yet one that is often overlooked. This step should be a formal process that may include written procedures and training and communication with everyone involved with the process. This includes staff members on off shifts, as well as staff in other departments who may be directly or indirectly affected by the changes. If necessary, post the standard work in the area where the process is performed. Make things as visual as possible and make it difficult to deviate from the standard. Remember, without standard work there is no continuous improvement.

CONCLUSION

Standard work is more than creating a standard of how work is to be performed. It is the heart and soul of Lean and it provides a platform for improvement.

By evaluating the current situation, identifying areas of opportunity, modifying the existing process, substantiating and enumerating improvements, and implementing the new standard of work, standard work initiates the lean transformation. Repeating the cycle for different processes perpetuates the lean transformation.

Standard work brings together lean tools and concepts in a structured approach that leads an organization to the benefits associated with a lean transformation. A lean transformation does not happen overnight. It takes years of dedication and commitment to the goal of eliminating non-value-added tasks in every area of the organization. The transformation takes place one project at a time. It is hard work, but the benefits are great and long lasting.

5S

Commonly misinterpreted as simply housekeeping, the implementation of 5S provides benefits that are far more than merely a neat and clean organization. If properly implemented, 5S will provide a solid foundation on which to build the lean organization. For this reason, it is commonly referred to as "the five pillars of the lean enterprise." Although housekeeping is its main focus, 5S also incorporates the standardization necessary to maintain the gains associated with any improvement initiative and the discipline needed to internalize those improvements.

The 5Ss are Japanese words that identify the five phases of implementation—Seri (say-ree), Seiton (say-tond), Seiso (say-so), Seiketsu (say-ket-soo), and Shitsuki (she-soo-kay). In English these words mean Organize, Orderliness, Cleanliness, Standardize, and Discipline. In order to maintain the 5S acronym used to describe this technique, five related English words beginning with the letter S have been adopted. In English, the five phases of implementation are *Sort, Straighten, Scrub, Standardize,* and *Sustain.*

The first three Ss relate specifically to housekeeping in the form of cleaning and organizing of the workplace. The fourth S focuses on establishing standard procedures, and the fifth S on developing the discipline necessary to the success of this initiative and all future lean initiatives. The last two, Standardize and Sustain, are beneficial in establishing the foundation on which to build the lean organization and creating a culture that will accept change. When coupled with other tools such as kanban (signal board) and visual controls, 5S becomes a powerful tool for eliminating non-value-added operations in the workplace. It also establishes a solid platform from which to launch future improvement initiatives. Kanban and visual controls will be discussed in the "Straighten" phase of this chapter.

When fully implemented, 5S eliminates the need to search for items, reduces the probability of errors, increases productivity, improves quality, ensures quicker response time, improves morale, and modifies the appearance of the department to convey a more professional image.

THE FIRST S – SEIRI – ORGANIZE – SORT

The focal point of the first S, Sort, is the elimination of unnecessary items in the workplace. As part of sorting, we clearly establish criteria for what is needed and what is not needed and separate these items accordingly. Items that are not needed are discarded or otherwise removed from the area. Needed items are sorted by frequency of use. Needed items fall into one of three categories: needed often, needed occasionally, or needed seldom (see Figure 6.1). Once sorted, frequently-used items are stored where they are easily accessible, preferably at point of use. Items used infrequently are stored further away but still readily available. Items that are rarely used are stored even further away, preferably outside of the area. The proper quantities of each item are determined during this phase; excessive quantities are relocated or discarded in order to maintain proper levels.

Sorting is essential to 5S because it eliminates clutter. Unneeded items can and will collect in the workplace over time. This accumulation happens so gradually that it often goes unnoticed. Eventually the cluttered work area becomes an obstacle course to be negotiated whenever an item is needed or work

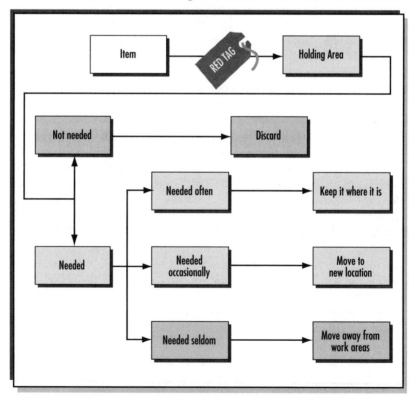

FIGURE 6.1   Flowchart for designating items in the sort phase.

must be performed. The department becomes increasingly crowded, valuable floor space disappears, staff must work around and climb over these obstructions, much time is wasted searching for items, and supplies and medications become prone to age-related deterioration. In some instances, shelves are built or lockers purchased to store unneeded items. There is no justification for the storage of unneeded items in the work area, yet this is a common solution for eliminating clutter in many organizations. In addition to causing non-value-added process steps, clutter hides problems such as missing items, defective equipment, or outdated medications and supplies. For these reasons, sorting is the logical first step in 5S and proper implementation is critical.

When implementing this phase, it may be helpful to recruit individuals from other areas or departments in the organization to assist in the sorting of items. These people will not have a sentimental attachment to items nor will they possess that "just in case" mentality created by past experience that makes people hoard supplies. Individuals not assigned to the area undergoing 5S have an objective attitude that may help ensure the success of the first phase of the project.

RED TAG STRATEGY

The method used to sort items in the workplace is known as the "Red Tag Strategy" (Hirano, 1989). Red tagging ensures that everyone has the opportunity to review items before they are categorized, moved, or discarded, thereby preventing the improper disposition (relocation or disposal) of items that may be needed by other individuals such as staff from the evening shift. In addition, red tagging limits the number of individuals authorized to order the disposition an item.

As the name implies, red-tagging consists of placing a red tag on items in the work area. It may be a professionally-printed red tag, a computer-generated red tag, or a simple white index card attached to the item with a piece of red tape. The tag itself is not important as long as it is clearly visible. More important than appearance is the information on the tag (see Figure 6.2). At a minimum, the information should include: the department, the date tagged, the name of the person tagging the item, the item description, the reason it is being tagged, disposition, the person who authorized the disposition, the asset code, and serial number. Because all items must be accounted for from a financial standpoint, these last two pieces of information are important for accounting purposes; be sure to involve accounting and purchasing during the sorting phase of 5S.

Red tagging begins with the placement of a red tag on any item of questionable need. This includes equipment, instruments, supplies, medications, paperwork, files, even signs and posters. Don't limit this effort to the general work area. Offices and work stations can benefit greatly from 5S as well. Try not to let frugality or sentimentality affect your judgment. If the

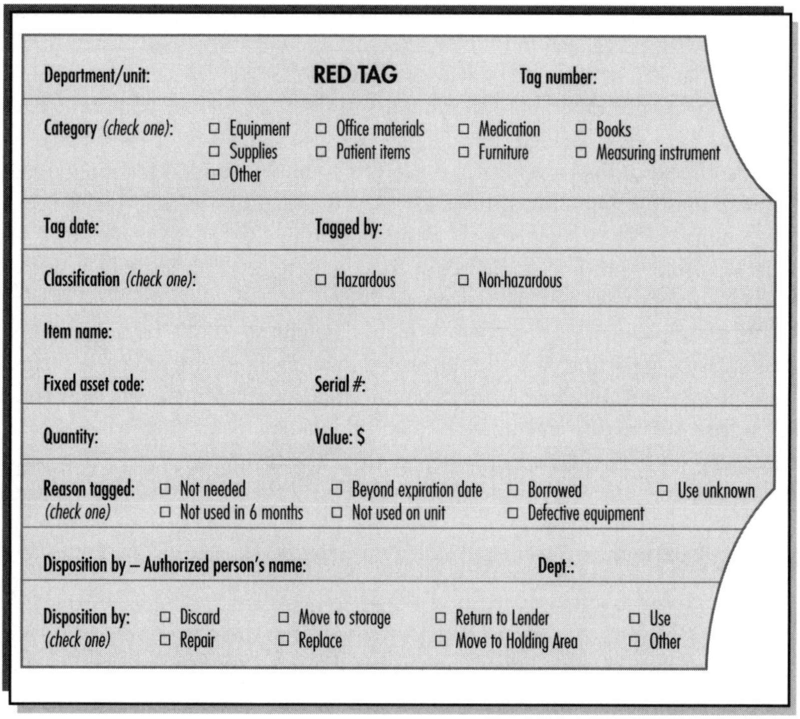

Department/unit:	**RED TAG**		Tag number:	
Category *(check one)*:	□ Equipment □ Supplies □ Other	□ Office materials □ Patient items	□ Medication □ Furniture	□ Books □ Measuring instrument

Tag date:	Tagged by:

Classification *(check one)*:	□ Hazardous	□ Non-hazardous

Item name:

Fixed asset code:	Serial #:

Quantity:	Value: $

Reason tagged: *(check one)*	□ Not needed □ Not used in 6 months	□ Beyond expiration date □ Not used on unit	□ Borrowed □ Defective equipment	□ Use unknown

Disposition by – Authorized person's name:	Dept.:

Disposition by: *(check one)*	□ Discard □ Repair	□ Move to storage □ Replace	□ Return to Lender □ Move to Holding Area	□ Use □ Other

FIGURE 6.2   A red tag.

item's value to the department is questionable, red tag it. Once the item is moved to a holding area, employees on all shifts have an opportunity to review the item and comment on its need before disposition.

An employee who has a concern regarding a specific item in the holding area may indicate that concern on the reverse side of the red tag for consideration by the person doing the disposition. After reviewing all the comments, authorized individuals submit items for disposition. Don't be too quick to dispose of items that have a discard disposition. Undamaged items and equipment may be sold, used by other departments, donated, or warehoused for future use. The goal of the sort phase is to remove unneeded items from the work area, not to throw away as much as possible regardless of condition.

Remove all red-tagged items from the area prior to starting the next phase of the 5S event. This will allow the team to get right to work on the next two phases.

THE SECOND S – SEITON – ORDERLINESS – STRAIGHTEN

Once unneeded items have been removed from an area, the next step is to organize those items that remain. Don't proceed to the second S unless you have successfully and completely implemented the first phase, sorting. Remember, organizing unneeded items is non-value added.

Skipping or improperly implementing the first phase and proceeding to the second phase will result in the creation of non-value-added work rather than the elimination of it. Only by combining the first two phases can the benefits of 5S be fully realized. Skipping steps gives the illusion of speed, but in reality it impedes improvement possibilities afforded by any lean initiative.

The second S focuses on the use of effective storage methods. Items should be arranged so that they are easy to find, easy to use, and easy to return to a designated location. The ultimate objective of 5S is that anyone, even someone not familiar with the area, should be able to find, use, and return what they need, when they need it. Things used frequently should be located closer to the user, while those infrequently or rarely needed may be placed further away.

Straightening provides the opportunity to be creative and imaginative and to have fun. The phrase "a place for everything and everything in its place" is the best description of what needs to be accomplished by straightening. Many techniques may be employed to achieve orderliness, such as shadow boards, color coding, and visual indicators.

The labeling of bins, shelves, cabinets and drawers should always be included during this phase of 5S. Staff should know what is in a cabinet or a drawer without having to open it and actually view the contents. Some organizations have gone so far as to install Plexiglas® doors on cabinets to allow viewing of contents without opening the cabinet door. Glass doors on cabinets were commonplace in hospitals and doctor's offices in years past, but the trend toward aesthetically pleasing furnishings changed that. Today, see-through doors once again eliminate the need to open and close cabinets. In addition, supplies are more likely to remain organized and orderly behind glass compared to supplies hidden behind an opaque door. The objective of straightening is to make an item both easy to find and easy to return to its proper location. Easy-to-find, easy-to-use, easy to-return is the mantra for this phase. Making something easy to find is only half the battle. If something is not returned to its designated area, the next person will not easily locate the item when it's needed again.

One creative way to organize the contents of drawers in desks or cabinets is to cut foam sheets to line drawers and then cut shapes in the foam to secure individual items. A strip of red tape placed at an angle across the bindings of a set of books or manuals is a simple, yet effective way to know, at a glance, if one is missing or out of place. These straightening techniques are shown in Figure 6.3 and Figure 6.4.

Two lean tools often used in conjunction with 5S are kanban and visual controls. The application and benefits of these two tools emerge during the straighten phase. Kanban can prove to be an indispensable tool for ensuring that the department always has sufficient supplies available for use. The opportunities for visual controls are limitless; they can eliminate huge amounts of waste.

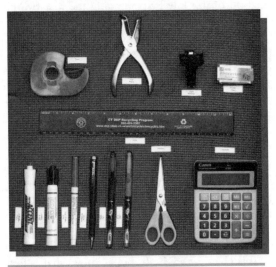

FIGURE 6.3   Example of a drawer organized with foam matting.

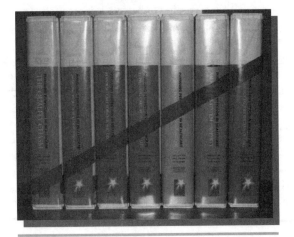

FIGURE 6.4   Example of colored tape used to ensure proper sequencing of manuals.

KANBAN

Kanban is a Japanese word that means sign board. A kanban signals that an item requires replenishing. The signal may take any form. It may be a card, a square painted on the floor, an empty bin, an alarm, or a light. The kanban should afford a quick response to a need, should provide precise information regarding what is needed, and should be inexpensive to implement. A sample kanban card is shown in Figure 6.5. Included on the card are the item name and part number, when and how many are needed, where the item is to be delivered, and a contact name and phone number. A picture of the item and a bar code are also helpful. The card can be color coded to indicate which department needs the item. This makes the cards easy to sort in the store room.

All kanbans need not be this elaborate. A card may be as simple as a part name and part number only. The detail on a kanban card is determined by the amount of information required by the person or department restocking the item. In many cases, other kanban signals may be better suited to the application than a card. Before implementing a kanban, be certain that the signal works for both the department using the item and the department replenishing it.

Regardless of form, all kanban signals work in a similar manner. When a stocked item is depleted to a predetermined level, the kanban (we will assume the card shown in Figure 6.5 for this example) is sent to the supplier indicating that the item must be replenished. When the supplier, in this case the storeroom, receives the card, they pick a box of fifty 30cc syringes from storage and schedule it for delivery to the unit no later than the following day. The min. and max. quantities indicated on the card are for use by the unit. If the level drops below 10, someone calls the storeroom immediately. There should never be more than two boxes of fifty 30cc syringes on the unit at one time. The storeroom returns the kanban card with the item when it is delivered. The card is kept with the item until it needs to be replenished again. This cycle is repeated whenever an item reaches the replenishing level, which is an estimate of how many items are required to ensure that the unit does not run out during the restocking period plus some small buffer to account for estimation errors, patient volume fluctuations, or emergency situations.

The storeroom should have its own kanban, called a withdrawal kanban, to indicate that a box of fifty 30cc syringes was pulled from stock and sent to the unit. This kanban signals the depletion of storeroom stock and the possible need for replenishment by the vendor.

Another example of a kanban is created by painting or taping two squares on the floor adjacent to each other, one yellow and one red. Placing full oxygen bottles within the yellow square and empty bottles within the red square lets the storeroom staff see at a glance if there is a need to replenish oxygen bottles.

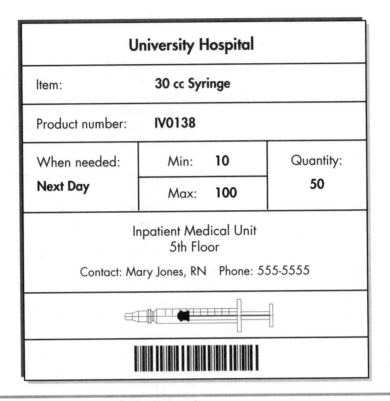

FIGURE 6.5 Example of a kanban card.

An empty bin may also be a kanban. Figure 6.6 shows a medication room that uses empty bins as the kanban. There are two bins for each item. Each bin has a label indicating item name and item number on one side and a bar code on the reverse. Needed items are taken only from the top bin until that bin is empty. The empty bin is then moved to the bottom; it becomes the kanban signaling the storeroom staff to replenish the item. The storeroom clerk removes the label and scans the barcode, ensuring that the items will be delivered on the next visit to the unit. This method ensures that there is always an ample supply of items on hand which are required for patient care. Items are easily located, the area is neat and orderly, and nurses are not burdened with the additional responsibility of ordering and keeping track of supplies. In addition, the kanban eliminates the duplication of orders resulting when several staff members order the same item.

These are only a few examples of kanbans. The possibilities are endless and they are all simple and inexpensive to implement. A kanban is a valuable tool to ensure that a department does not run out of parts or supplies. It also prevents the expiration of supplies and medications.

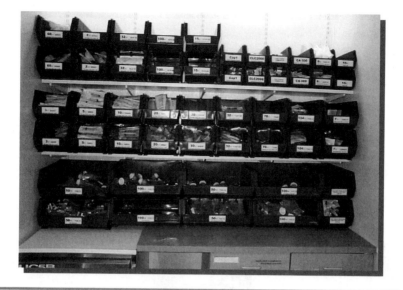

FIGURE 6.6   Empty-bin kanban system.

When setting up a kanban, it's important to be familiar with the different kinds of inventory systems. The three most commonly used inventory systems are: FIFO (First-In, First-Out), LIFO (Last-In, First-Out), and Weighted Average. These systems, originally established for accounting purposes, relate to the value of the inventory based on the purchase of raw materials. Relative to a kanban, it is important to be familiar only with FIFO and LIFO, and then only from the standpoint of expiration or spoilage. In the supermarket, the dairy display case is loaded from the rear and customers take the milk from the front. This is a FIFO system. It ensures that the oldest milk is purchased first so that it does not go out of date before it is sold. When pizzas are stocked in the freezer section of the supermarket, the newer items are stacked on top of the older items (unless the stock clerk rotates the stock). This is an example of a LIFO system. Figure 6.7 provides a pictorial representation of both FIFO and LIFO inventory systems. LIFO is only desirable from an accounting viewpoint and should be avoided when setting up a kanban.

A kanban may be useful for surgical kits, equipment, medications, and forms. It may also be used to improve patient flow. By incorporating kanbans, the likelihood of running out of an item can be reduced to zero. The non-value-added activity associated with searching for and obtaining items can be totally eliminated. This is the basic philosophy behind Just-In-Time (JIT). JIT means having what is needed, when it's needed, in the quantity needed, every time it's needed. By implementing kanbans, this can be accomplished.

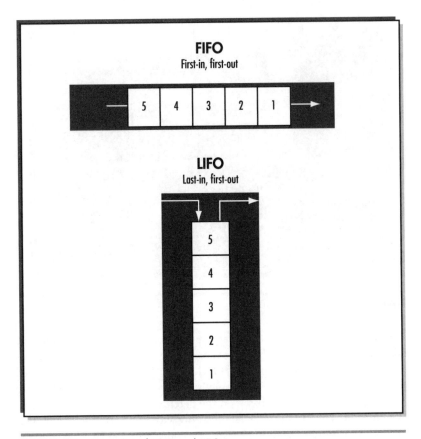

FIGURE 6.7 Examples of FIFO and LIFO inventory systems.

VISUAL CONTROLS

A visual control is simply a method used to share information nonverbally. When visual controls are properly implemented, everyone is aware of the current situation. They understand the work process and they know the schedule. Abnormalities readily become obvious. Dr. Gwendolyn D. Galsworth, the author of *The Power Of Visual Information Sharing On The Shop Floor For The Small Manufacturer*, describes visual controls as "self-explaining, self ordering, self regulating, and self-improving—where what is supposed to happen does happen, on time, every time, day or night" (Galsworth, 1995).

The scoreboard at a baseball game is a visual control. Although the action takes place on the field, someone who wants to know what is going on looks at the scoreboard. It provides much more information than just the score. It tells the fans in which inning the runs were scored, how many hits each team got, and how many errors they made. It tells which team is batting, which player is at bat, how many balls and how many strikes have been recorded. Using visuals, the scoreboard announces the current situation (self-explaining), how far the game has progressed (self-ordering), and which team is ahead or behind (self-regulating). It also identifies abnormal conditions (self-improving). The scoreboard provides the same information to everyone, keeps the team focused on what is important, and lets everyone know what must happen in order to win the game.

There are four categories of visual control:

1. Visual indicators

2. Visual signals

3. Visual controls

4. Visual guarantees

Visual indicators, the simplest form of visual control, include things such as signs on the door of a patient's room or stickers on the patient's medical record indicating special needs such as "No B/P or venipuncture, right arm," or "Anticoagulants, hold all needle sites 5 minutes minimum." Visual indicators are inexpensive and easy to implement and offer a myriad of possibilities.

The next category, visual signals, includes lights and alarms. A nurse-call light is a perfect example of a visual signal. Visual signals do not necessarily require expensive systems. The colored tabs separating the different sections of a manual are inexpensive visual signals.

In the third category are visual controls that limit actions. For example, by providing a bin for storage of a certain part, the department ensures that excess parts will not be delivered to the unit. The mail-box-top sharps container is a visual control. When the bucket is full, the top does not open to receive additional items and the container must be replaced.

Last is the visual guarantee, which eliminates the possibility of error. The quick-connect fittings for different gases in the operating room, a different size and color for each gas, eliminate the possibility of using the wrong gas.

The possibilities are limitless for implementing visuals controls. Use them whenever possible. Creating a visual workplace eliminates the need to search for items and eliminates waiting because information is readily available, accurate, complete, and reliable.

THE THIRD S – SEISO – CLEANLINESS – SCRUB

The third S is dedicated to cleaning. This is obviously a much bigger job in a manufacturing environment than in a hospital, but dirt, stains, and debris do develop in hospitals. Windows, equipment, light fixtures, and ceiling tiles routinely need cleaning, but don't limit your attention to only these areas. Focus on walls and floor, desk tops and counters, sinks, carts, and anything else that requires cleaning. If you can't get something clean, paint it, replace it, or cover it. The workplace should be clean and bright, a place where people enjoy working. The Environmental Services department is probably already doing an excellent job, so this S should not require a major effort.

Try to think of ways to prevent messes from happening in the first place. For example, expelling air from a syringe may result in medication being squirted on the walls and ceiling. This can produce unsightly stains. A Plexiglas® shield at the medication station will prevent medication from reaching the walls and ceiling. The inexpensive Plexiglas® can be scheduled for replacement at regular intervals.

THE FOURTH S – SEIKETSU –
STANDARDIZE – STABILIZE

Backsliding happens very slowly and may go unnoticed for long periods of time. Dust and dirt begin to accumulate. Items, books, and equipment are left lying around rather than being put back where they came from. Spills and messes are left for someone else to clean up. Before you know it, you're back to square one. This is where the benefits of the fourth S, standardize, can be realized. This phase is crucial to the success of the 5S improvement effort and success with this phase will carry over to other lean initiatives.

Standardization helps to maintain the gains achieved by implementation of the first three Ss. Because everyone must be responsible for maintaining the benefits, everyone must know what is expected. Communication is critical during this phase. Everyone must be educated regarding kanban, visual controls, and general housekeeping.

Photographs of a medication room before and after 5S are shown in Figure 6.8. The results of the first three Ss are obvious. Unneeded items have been removed from the area and remaining items have been organized. The room is neat, clean, and orderly. The room is brighter, there is no clutter, items are easy to find, and there is plenty of available work surface. These benefits will result in fewer errors, better efficiency, and a safer work environment. Unless procedures are standardized to maintain these benefits, it will be only a matter of time before the medication room once again looks like the "before" photograph.

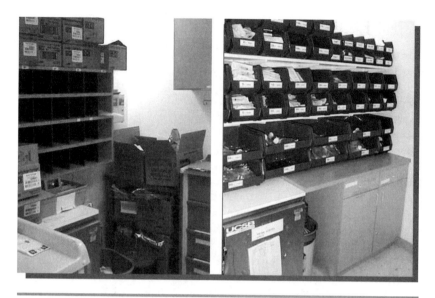

FIGURE 6.8 Medication room before and after 5S.

The staff must be instructed to remove items from the top bin only, and to switch bins when the top one becomes empty. If that training does not occur, the kanban will not work. Unless the stockroom clerk is instructed that an empty bin is a signal to replenish an item, the kanban will not be successful. The success or failure of improvement initiatives relies on everyone knowing what needs to be done and doing it. This is accomplished by standardization. Keep it simple. Do not devise elaborate and complicated procedures for standardization. The more complicated the standard, the less likely it is to be followed and the less likely you will maintain the gains.

Imagine the medication room without standards. Items would be removed from both bins. The storeroom would replenish items only when a request was made by someone on the unit, and that request would always require immediate attention. Items would end up in the wrong bins. Unopened cases would be stacked wherever there was room available. Slowly but surely, the medication room would begin to look as it did before the 5S implementation.

Success of a 5S initiative cannot be delegated to an individual or group of individuals. Everyone must be held accountable for doing what is expected. Management must take appropriate action when staff are not doing their parts. A reminder of the goals will usually bring people on board and will provide more success than reprimanding the individual. 5S is everyone's responsibility.

THE FIFTH S – SHITSUKI – DISCIPLINE – SUSTAIN

The fifth and final phase of 5S deals with developing a habit. Research tells us that it takes twenty-one days to form a habit. That's three weeks. You will know a habit has been formed when it feels uncomfortable to do things "wrong." Everyone should feel uncomfortable failing to put items back in the drawer, neglecting to refill the paper towel dispenser, ignoring trash accumulating in the corner, hoarding supplies "just in case," or doing anything else not consistent with the goal of maintaining a 5S environment.

No matter how well the first four Ss are implemented, the benefits will be lost without discipline. The natural tendency is to return to the status quo. Sustaining the gains is, without a doubt, the most difficult phase of 5S. The area may be clean and organized, standards may be in place, everyone may be aware of the standards, but without discipline, the gains will surely be lost.

The fifth S, sustain, is the responsibility of management. It cannot be delegated and is best taught by example.

KEYS TO SUCCESS WITH 5S

- The first step in any improvement initiative should be communication. Tell everyone about 5S and explain why it is important to the organization. Conduct training sessions, issue memos, post signs, do whatever is necessary to ensure that everyone is aware of the activity that is about to take place.

- Obtain commitment from management to provide the resources necessary to successfully implement the first three Ss and the leadership necessary to achieve the last two.

- Use as many visuals as possible. Look for opportunities to create kanbans. Be creative, and have fun.

- Remember that the goal of 5S is twofold, to clean and organize the workplace thereby eliminating sources of non-value-added work. More importantly, however, 5S establishes the foundation for the lean organization. Make the foundation strong and solid and you will realize the benefits as the organization builds upon that foundation.

MISTAKE PROOFING

At Toyota, they call it poka-yoke, which is derived from two Japanese words. Yokeru means to avoid; poka means errors. Hence, poka-yoke means to avoid errors. Mistakes and the defects they cause are twice as costly to an organization when evaluated from a lean perspective. If a process laden with non-value-adding operations generates an error, it becomes necessary to repeat the process and all it's non-value-adding components. There is also the non-value-added activity directly associated with the defect or error and its correction.

To better understand mistake proofing, it is important to distinguish between a mistake and a defect. A mistake, as defined by the Institute of Medicine, is "the failure of a planned action to be completed as intended or the use of a wrong plan to achieve an aim" (Committee on Quality of Healthcare in America, Institute of Medicine, 2000). Defects are the end result of a mistake. For example, not checking for drug interaction and compatibility before administering the drug to a patient is a mistake. The reaction a patient experiences as a result of the adverse drug event is a defect.

Defects and the mistakes that cause them are costly to hospitals. Failure to address deficiencies that result in medical errors within the care delivery process costs hospitals an estimated $17 billion to $29 billion per year nationwide. Monetary costs are not the only penalty hospitals pay for medical errors. Hospitals must also endure the negative effect on the staff morale and the loss of community trust (Committee on Quality of Healthcare in America, Institute of Medicine, 2000). There is one simple fact, however, that cannot be denied. Everyone makes mistakes. It was Teddy Roosevelt who said, "The only man who makes no mistakes is the man who never does anything." Common mistakes in our society result from confusing directions or instructions, errors in calculations, distractions, carelessness, rushing, and improper training, among other things. Mistake proofing, however, has the very real capability of diminishing or even eradicating the defects resulting from mistakes in hospitals.

Wrong site surgeries, adverse drug events, improper transfusion, falls, mixed lab specimens, and mistaken patient identities occur in hospitals every day, so the opportunities for mistake proofing in healthcare are limitless. Hospitals must not accept mistakes as a consequence of the complexity of the care delivery system. Instead, having conceded that people make mistakes, the organization must put in place devices and systems that will prevent mistakes or detect them before they result in defects.

Mistake proofing uses devices or methods to prevent, detect, or minimize the effects of mistakes. These need not be expensive software packages or costly equipment. On the contrary, many mistake-proofing devices and methods are simple, inexpensive, and effective. Developed through the creativity and resolve of an improvement team assigned to a project, they offer options for preventing and detecting errors.

There are three levels of mistake proofing. Level 1 prevents a mistake from ever occurring. Naturally this is the most desirable level, but it is not always possible. Level 2 detects the occurrence of a mistake before it results in a defect. Level 3, the least desirable, detects that a mistake has resulted in a defect but prevents the defect from causing irreparable damage.

Developing a mistake-proofing device or system is accomplished by means of a five-step method that involves defining the mistake or defect in detail, identifying the conditions that may lead to the mistake, conducting a root-cause analysis, generating ideas to eliminate future mistakes, and developing and implementing the device or method (see Figure 7.1).

DEFINE THE MISTAKE OR DEFECT

The first step in mistake proofing is to define the mistake or defect in detail. Document specifically what it is. When does it occur? When does it not occur? Where did it take place and where was it detected? Who identified the mistake or defect? Who made the mistake, and was this the result of deviation from the standard operating procedure? If there was a deviation from the standard, what

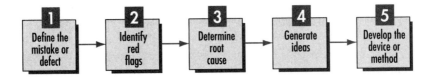

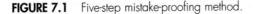

FIGURE 7.1   Five-step mistake-proofing method.

was it? Why was the standard not followed? How was the mistake or defect detected? Why did it happen? This last question requires that the team keep an open mind. Although the cause of the problem may seem obvious, the real reason for an error may be rooted much deeper in the process. Jumping to conclusions may lead to superficial solutions that only mask the problem, allowing the real cause of the error or defect to go undetected and resulting in a serious or even catastrophic incident. This complicates the problem rather than eliminating it. Any information or data relative to the mistake or defect should be gathered and analyzed at this time. Have there been previous incidents? How many? Is there a trend? Where did they happen? When did they happen? How and by whom were they detected? Formulating and asking the right questions is a fundamental practice in any problem-solving exercise. Be sure to get all the facts before proceeding. Assume nothing.

RED FLAGS

A condition that provokes the likelihood of a mistake is referred to as a red flag. These are conditions inherent in the process. There is no all-inclusive list of red flags to cover every situation. The flags will be different for every process. There are, however, several that are common and it is worthwhile to be aware of them. Post a list of these common red flags where it is easily seen by the mistake-proofing team. They will find it a handy reference during the event.

Repetition is the first red flag condition. Whenever routine tasks are repeated over and over, there is a high likelihood that mistakes will occur. Repetitious processes are better suited to robots than people. A person may be distracted or become bored; loss of concentration can result in mistakes. Over time, workers become very comfortable with the tasks necessary to complete a process or operation and are apt to miss or overlook a step. If a repetitious process must be conducted at an accelerated pace, the chance of a mistake occurring is even greater.

Another red-flag condition occurs when an operation or process is conducted infrequently. Unfamiliarity with a process provides as many opportunities for mistakes as overfamiliarity caused by repetition. Making assumptions about new equipment or a new terminology can lead to mistakes. Often people try to remember the process steps rather than refer to the standard for direction. Relying on memory to execute a process that is performed infrequently provides a huge opportunity for mistakes.

Similarity of patient names and medications with similar names or appearance should also raise a red flag. This situation is common in healthcare. For example, consider Celebrex,™ a drug that provides pain relief, and Cerebyx,™ an anticonvulsant prescribed for the treatment of seizures. These could easily be confused.

Combining red-flag conditions will increase the likelihood of mistakes. Combine similarity with repetition, for example, and the likelihood of errors increases significantly.

A sequenced process is another red flag. Whenever a process must be performed in a specific sequence there is the potential to miss a task, repeat a task, or perform a task out of sequence.

Other red flags include high patient volume, poorly defined standards, and environmental conditions such as poor lighting. Red-flag conditions must be highlighted and acted upon in order to eliminate the occurrence of mistakes and subsequent defects.

ROOT CAUSE ANALYSIS

The next and most important step in the mistake-proofing process is the root cause analysis (RCA). Techniques for determining root cause range from the simple Five Whys to the more structured Failure Mode and Effects Analysis (FMEA).

Don't overlook the Five Whys (covered in Chapter 5: Standard Work) because of the simplicity of the method. No matter how simple or complex the method, the result of an RCA is identification of the root cause of the problem only, not the solution. If the root cause of the problem can be determined simply by utilizing the Five Whys and the team exhibits a high level of confidence with the results, then by all means use it. Employing a more complex RCA method will provide no additional benefit; it may actually be non-value-added under some circumstances.

A crucial undertaking in any root-cause analysis is the validity of the information. Current and accurate information is essential to successfully determining the root cause of an error. Most of the time spent in root-cause analysis will be to collect information and verify it. Take the time necessary to collect new and accurate information. Do not use information from last year, last quarter, or even last month. Always gather current information that reflects the situation surrounding the mistake or defect.

CAUSE-AND-EFFECT DIAGRAM

A cause-and-effect (C&E) diagram is a more structured approach to determining the root cause of a mistake. The C&E diagram, or fishbone diagram, was developed by Professor Kaoru Ishikawa of Tokyo University in Japan. It is sometimes referred to as the Ishikawa diagram.

The C&E diagram identifies the inputs or potential causes of a single output or effect. The work that takes place every day in a hospital may be divided into six distinct categories. Each day services are provided in response to doctor's orders (instruction) using supplies and pharmaceuticals (materials) or equipment (machinery) so that the hospital staff (people) can provide the necessary care/service in accordance with established procedures (methods) within the hospital setting (environment). These six categories make up the six branches of the C&E diagram (see Figure 7.2). Once the branches are identified, follow these steps to construct the diagram:

1. Before beginning, be sure everyone agrees on the effect selected for the study.

2. Brainstorm possible causes (primary causes) and draw them as extensions to the appropriate branch of the diagram.

3. For the primary causes on each branch, ask why they are occurring (secondary causes). Draw these secondary causes as extensions to the primary causes (see Figure 7.2). The lines are for illustrative purposes only; for your own C&E diagram, draw lines for each primary and secondary cause as they are identified.

4. Analyze the causes. Look for problems that occur in more than one category.

5. Prioritize and identify those causes that are most likely to be the root cause of the stated effect.

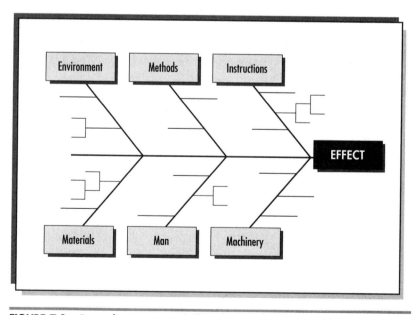

FIGURE 7.2   Frame for a cause-and-effect diagram.

Remember that the C&E diagram does not provide a solution, nor does any other RCA technique. It does, however, help to organize thoughts with a structured process and present all possible causes. It is an effective technique for generating theories about the root cause(s) of a problem. The C&E diagram may identify more than one cause for the mistake or error (effect). The team may decide to address all, some, or only one of the causes. This is totally acceptable. It is better to generate and implement a device or method to address a single cause of the problem than to declare the problem too complex and put it off for another time.

Use a whiteboard or large sheets of paper taped to a wall in the front of the room to construct the cause-and-effect diagram. This will help create a team focus. Use Post-It Notes™ to insert primary and secondary causes on the diagram. This will allow you to make changes without crossing out or erasing.

GENERATING IDEAS

In most cases, brainstorming is the tool of choice for generating ideas. (Brainstorming is covered in detail in Chapter 5: Standard Work.) Try brainstorming to generate ideas that will prevent mistakes from occurring, that will identify mistakes before they cause defects, or that will minimize the effect of defects. This is a time to be creative. Encourage all ideas. Never reject an idea as frivolous or inappropriate. An idea that seems irrelevant may trigger another idea that leads to a solution. Inappropriate ideas may be eliminated later, during the list-reduction phase of the brainstorming exercise.

Once ideas have been generated, they must be categorized and prioritized. Use the affinity diagram (categorize) and the prioritization matrix (prioritize) to accomplish these tasks.

AFFINITY DIAGRAM

After brainstorming to generate ideas and using list-reduction techniques to clarify unclear issues, eliminate duplicates, and remove the irrelevant, inappropriate, or not feasible ideas, you must organize what remains on the list. The affinity diagram helps you organize ideas by making logical connections between issues.

As the facilitator of the brainstorming process records ideas on the flip chart, a team member should write each idea on an individual Post-it™ note. During the list-reduction phase, remove notes for any ideas that have been eliminated from the list. Then post remaining notes on a large and easily accessible wall in a random fashion to begin the affinity diagram. Team members may go to the wall and arrange the notes into groupings of similar items. Ideally this is done in silence, without any discussion. A team member who disagrees with the placement of a note is free to move it to a more appropriate location. A note that does not fit into a grouping may stand alone as an orphan. Having arranged the notes, the team may now return to their seats and begin to discuss the best name for each group. Chosen names are written on Post-it notes of another color and placed at the top of the appropriate grouping. Once the ideas have been categorized and the categories named, the team will prioritize groupings relative to which ideas will have the greatest impact on reducing or eliminating mistakes. What has been created through this process is called an affinity diagram.

PRIORITIZATION MATRIX

As the name implies, this matrix prioritizes ideas based on their importance to the organization relative to established decisive factors. To accomplish this, ideas are scored against a set of key criteria. The scores are weighted relative to their importance and totaled for each criterion.

To construct a prioritization matrix (see Figure 7.3), the team will develop criteria upon which each idea will be evaluated. For the example illustrated, the criteria for evaluation are cost of implementation, ease of implementation, the level of the proposed mistake-proofing device or method, and the time required to implement the device or method. Each criterion is then assigned a numerical range for scoring purposes. For example, the category "Device level" scores a 9 if the device prevents a mistake from occurring, a 3 if it detects a mistake before it becomes a defect, and a 1 if it minimizes the impact of the defect. Using values such as 1, 3, and 9, or 0, 5, and 10 will reduce the occurrence of total scores that are too close to differentiate.

The next step is to weight each criterion based on its importance to the organization. (Note the shaded area of the matrix in Figure 7.3). In this example, the cost to implement is not a major concern; "Cost to implement" is assigned a lower weighting. Conversely, having the device or method in place as soon as possible is important; "Time to implement" is assigned a higher weight. At this point, previously generated and evaluated ideas recorded in the left hand column are given a score in each of the categories. The score is multiplied by the weight, the four products are summed, and the totals are recorded in the appropriate column. The idea with the highest score receives the highest priority and should be chosen for implementation. The total for idea 1 was calculated as follows:

$$(1 \times 9) + (1.5 \times 3) + (2 \times 1) + (1 \times 3) = 18.5$$

Mistake-Proofing Prioritization Matrix

Weight	Cost to implement 1 – High 3 – Mid Range 9 – Low 1	Ease of implementation 1 – Difficult 3 – Doable 9 – Easy 1.5	Device level 1 – Minimizes 3 – Detects 9 – Prevents 2	Time to implement 1 – Long 3 – Reasonable 9 – Quick 1	Total
Idea 1	9	3	1	3	18.5
Idea 2	3	3	9	9	34.5
Idea 3	1	1	3	1	9.5

FIGURE 7.3 Mistake-proofing prioritization matrix.

DEVELOPING THE DEVICE OR METHOD

The final step in the mistake-proofing process involves the development and implementation of the device or method that will detect or prevent the mistake from occurring again. Although it may seem that this final step would occur almost automatically, it is frequently the most difficult to accomplish. Priorities change, emergencies arise, and initiatives are often put aside and forgotten. To prevent this loss of momentum it's vital that the team leader, with the support of management, track and follow up on the the selected priority. The tool utilized to track the progress of incomplete tasks is the Continuous Improvement (CI) to-do list, which is essentially an action-item list that visually displays progress. The CI to-do list highlights an incomplete task, the person responsible for it, the date it was due, and progress toward its completion (see Figure 7.4). To be effective, the form must be plainly visible to everyone in the area where the work is performed, for example the medication room or the nurse's station. As progress occurs, the sectioned circle associated with each task is filled in to indicate 25, 50, 75, and 100 percent completion. This allows management and everyone else to see, at a glance, that progress is being made toward the development and implementation of the mistake-proofing device or method. The CI to-do list is a simple visual indicator that helps keep assigned tasks from falling by the wayside.

MISTAKE-PROOFING WORKSHEET

The mistake-proofing worksheet shown in Figure 7.5 is a useful tool for guiding a team through the five-step process. The facilitator should enlarge the form and place it on the wall in the front of the room so everyone on the improvement team can view it at the same time. The form follows the steps outlined in this chapter.

Continuous Improvement To-Do List

Team: _____ Date: _____

No.	Problem/issue/opportunity	Countermeasure	Person responsible	Date/time due	% complete
					100 / 75 ⊘ 25 / 50
					100 / 75 ⊘ 25 / 50
					100 / 75 ⊘ 25 / 50
					100 / 75 ⊘ 25 / 50
					100 / 75 ⊘ 25 / 50
					100 / 75 ⊘ 25 / 50
					100 / 75 ⊘ 25 / 50
					100 / 75 ⊘ 25 / 50
					100 / 75 ⊘ 25 / 50
					100 / 75 ⊘ 25 / 50

Lean Hospitals
Bringing Lean to Healthcare

FIGURE 7.4 Continuous improvement to-do list.

Mistake-Proofing Worksheet

Is this a mistake or defect?   ☐ Mistake   ☐ Defect

Description: _____

_____

_____

Where_____	**When**_____	**Who**_____
Detected:	Date:	Detected:
Occurred:	Time:	Made:

Describe the situation leading to the mistake/defect:_____

_____

_____

_____

Was there a deviation from the standards?   ☐ Yes   ☐ No
If yes, describe:_____

Information regarding previous occurrences: _____

_____

_____

Red Flag conditions: _____

Root Cause 1:	Root Cause 2:	Root Cause 3:

Device or method for root cause 1:_____

_____

Device or method for root cause 2:_____

_____

Device or method for root cause 3:_____

_____

FIGURE 7.5   Mistake-proofing worksheet.

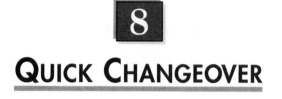

8

QUICK CHANGEOVER

I n manufacturing, changing over an assembly line or a piece of equipment to accommodate the production of a different product often involves a significant amount of time. Since lean focuses on meeting customer demands, the ability to quickly change over from one product to another is essential to maintaining flow. This concept is as valid in healthcare as it is in manufacturing. The ability to change over from one patient to the next, from one test to the next, and from one operating room to the next is critical to maintaining flow. Quick changeover (or setup reduction) has the potential to increase revenue, reduce costs, enhance customer satisfaction, and ensure the unobstructed flow of a process. Like most lean tools and concepts, quick changeover requires ingenuity and persistence on the part of the improvement team, and the rewards are often impressive. It is not uncommon to see change-over time reductions as high as 80 percent.

A changeover initiative for CT Scans at a small community hospital resulted in an 82 percent reduction in the time required for changeover from one patient to the next, allowing the hospital to conduct twice as many scans on any given day. This, in turn, eliminated backlogs and significantly increased revenue. The changeover reduction initiative permitted maximum utilization of the CT scanner by increasing the machines uptime.

About 1950, Shigeo Shingo, a pioneer in the development of the Toyota Production System, began to study the effects of improvement in changeover times in manufacturing. He developed a set-up time reduction system that he called SMED, an acronym for single minute exchange of die. The basic goal of SMED was the ability to change over from one product to the next in less than ten minutes. Shingo realized that there are two fundamentally different types of changeover operations. He categorized these as "internal" times and "external" times (Shingo, 1983). Internal time accrues while the machine or resource is not running. This is essentially lost money, since a machine only generates revenue when it is in use. External time accrues while the machine is running. Minimizing or eliminating internal time or, if necessary, converting it to external time maximizes machine utilization. Keep in mind the goal is not to maximize external time, only to minimize or eliminate internal time.

CHANGEOVER TIME

The starting point for any quick-changeover project is to clearly define when the changeover time begins and when it ends. This may seem obvious, but changeover time does not begin when a patient leaves the room and it does not end when the next patient is called. Changeover time begins the moment the machine is turned off; it ends when the machine is turned back on to provide the service for which it was intended, error free. For example, if it is necessary to conduct a trial run before actually using the machine for its intended purpose, the trial run must be included in the changeover time. The trial run is categorized as external time since the machine is running, but this is non-value-added time. In this example, every effort is made to eliminate the need for a trial run. Ideally, a machine should be ready to operate error free, first time and every time. Trial runs are non-value-added activities; make every effort to eliminate them.

Once changeover beginning and ending times have been clearly defined, changeover analysis can begin. This analysis is conducted using the Changeover Analysis Worksheet shown in Figure 8.1.

PROCESS FOR CHANGEOVER ANALYSIS

1. Identify all tasks conducted from the moment the machine is turned off until it is turned back on and providing the service for which it was intended, error free. Document these tasks on the worksheet under the column heading "Element/Task Description." As with time observations, a video camera is useful for observing a changeover.

2. Classify and document each of the tasks identified in step 1 as either internal or external. Remember, internal means the task is performed while the machine is not running. External tasks are performed while the machine is running.

3. Determine the time required to complete each task and the cumulative changeover cycle time. Record these times on the worksheet under the appropriate column headings.

4. Associate each task with one or more of the following categories:
   a. Preparation (P) – These are tasks performed to prepare the patient, product, or machine for test. This includes tasks such as obtaining supplies, verifying orders, starting IVs, registering a patient, or explaining the procedure.

Changeover Analysis Worksheet

Machine: _____   Date: _____

Step	Time		Class Before	Element/Task Description	Before				Amount of			After Time	After			
	Cumulative	Task	Int/Ext		Category by				Move to External	Reduced	Eliminated		Category by			
					P	L	A	S					P	L	A	S
TOTALS																

CATEGORIES: P – Preparation   L – Loading & Unloading   A – Align & Adjust   S – Secure

Number of steps moved to external: _____   Time moved to external: _____   Number of steps reduced: _____   Time reduced: _____   Number of steps eliminated: _____   Time eliminated: _____

FIGURE 8.1   Changeover analysis worksheet.

b. Loading and Unloading (L) – This category includes the tasks of loading and unloading of patients, product, or supplies. Examples of this category include moving the patient from a stretcher to an exam table, loading or unloading specimens in a blood chemistry analyzer, and assembling a special MRI procedure coil.

c. Alignment and Adjustment (A) – These are steps required to position the patient or product. Adjusting the height of a table, lining up a beam, or positioning specimen containers so that bar codes face out for reading are all operations that are considered alignment or adjustment.

d. Secure (S) – These are tasks that require fastening, latching, clamping, strapping, or any other means of keeping the patient or product from moving during the test.

5. For each task, brainstorm ideas to eliminate or minimize internal times or convert them to external times. Converting internal operations to external operations provides an opportunity for reducing setup time when tasks cannot be eliminated. Any task that does not require the machine to be shut down should be conducted while the machine is running.

6. For all operations, but especially internal operations, devise ways to reduce the amount of time required to complete the task. Eliminating the need to make adjustments can significantly reduce the time required. Consider methods to quickly secure products or patients that do not include cranking, buckling, threading or turning a screw,. Using guide pins or positioning blocks to assure quick and accurate alignment can also reduce task times. Conduct operations in a logical sequence that will minimize excess motion and maximize efficiency.

7. Verify the necessity of every task. If an operation is not absolutely required, consider eliminating it. Many tasks are performed simply because "that's the way we've always done it."

8. Quantify improvements and record results on the worksheet in the appropriate sections.

9. Develop standard work (see Chapter 5). Remember, without standard work there is no continuous improvement. Establish a standard procedure and ensure that it is being followed.

PREPARATION TIME

Tasks required to prepare a patient or product for test must never be conducted while the machine sits idle. These operations can and should be completed while the machine is being utilized on a prior patient or product. The only exception to this occurs when volumes are too low to provide a steady stream of patients or products, or when the test is required infrequently or sporadically. Whenever possible, make every attempt to schedule equipment use to create a constant and steady flow.

A sequence of events taken to complete a CT scan changeover might be described as follows:

- Scan ends; machine is turned off

- IV is remove from patient

- Patient is removed from scan bed

- Patient is brought out of the CT scan room

- Next patient is brought into the CT scan room

- Patient ID is verified

- Procedure is explained to patient

- Physicians orders are verified

- IV is started on patient

- Patient is placed on scan bed

- CT scan is turned on; machine begins scan

These steps are considered internal time (non-value-added) if conducted while the machine is not running. A changeover reduction analysis would immediately highlight the fact that ascertaining ID, explaining the procedure, verifying orders, and starting the IV are all preparation tasks that could be performed while the machine is in use for another patient, effectively reclassifying them as external. Now internal, or non-value-added, time is reduced to include only the time required to remove the IV and transport the first patient from the room. The next patient is then brought in, placed on the table and scanning is begun. Even removing the IV from the first patient could be done externally. The changeover procedure now has fewer internal operations.

- Scan ends; machine is turned off

- Patient is removed from scan bed

- Patient is brought out of the CT scan room

- Next patient is brought into the CT scan room

- Patient is placed on scan bed

- CT Scan is turned on; machine begins scan

Converting internal preparation operations to external operations reduces the number of operations required by more than 50 percent. This, in turn, reduces the amount of changeover time by more than 80 percent.

LOADING AND UNLOADING TIME

Loading and unloading fall into a category that is almost always conducted internally. The time required to load and unload the machine with a patient or product usually appears insignificant relative to other categories in the changeover process. Even so, loading and unloading the machine, in the most efficient and effective way, should be the only operations conducted internally. Removing one patient from the scan bed and positioning the next scheduled patient should, ideally, be the entire changeover procedure. This is not always realistic, but minimizing the time required for performing the tasks related to the other operation categories, or eliminating those tasks altogether, is central to a successful changeover reduction project.

ALIGNMENT AND ADJUSTMENT TIME

Whenever alignments or adjustments are mentioned in connection with a changeover procedure, a flag should go up indicating an opportunity for improvement. Guide pins, stop blocks, and easily readable and visible scales are only a few of the options available to reduce the time required to adjust and align equipment. Tasks in this category are often repeated again and again as a result of trial-and-error positioning. They should be performed only once. Re-adjustment and re-alignment are non-value-added tasks that should be totally eliminated from the setup procedures. If possible, the patient or product should be aligned as part of the loading procedure. Any adjustments required after loading the patient or product are strictly non-value-added and must be minimized or eliminated.

A trial run comes under this heading since the purpose of the trial run is to verify the positioning or alignment of the equipment being used. Trial runs can consume significant amounts of time, especially if several runs are required before the desired condition is established and the test can proceed. The success rate of a trial run is usually dependent on the skill, knowledge and experience of the person conducting the test. To reduce the number of trial runs, it is necessary to minimize the number of adjustments required at each changeover. It should never be necessary to conduct more than one trial run.

SECURING TIME

The final category deals with securing the patient or product in the machine. Minimizing the time required to do this can make changeover much faster and easier. The many varieties of quick-clamping mechanisms available allow you to secure a patient or product safely, quickly, and reliably. Avoid using screw-type devices whenever possible, especially any that require more than a quarter turn to be engaged. Also avoid buckles on straps used to secure patients. Restraints made with Velcro straps are quicker, safer, and equally effective.

It's often necessary to secure a patient's extremities to minimize movement during a test. Many times this also requires adjustment and alignment. Developing standardized fixtures will reduce the need for adjustments and alignment for securing extremities.

CONCLUSION

Reducing changeover time can significantly improve flow and enhance the quality and pace at which services are provided to customers. These techniques should not be limited to equipment changeover. Changeover analysis projects in operating rooms, special procedure rooms, even inpatient rooms after discharge can provide huge benefits.

Remember the two basic concepts of quick changeover: Conduct as many of the changeover operations as possible while the machine is running, and minimize the steps and the time required to complete each step.

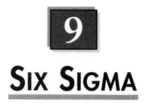

SIX SIGMA

There was a time when Lean and Six Sigma were believed to be opposing methodologies. In the past few years, however, the marriage of these two methodologies has given rise to a new concept, Lean-Sigma. This new idea is rapidly gaining popularity. Six Sigma is more of a quality improvement methodology while Lean is more a process improvement methodology, but the two are complimentary and can be implemented simultaneously. The logical order of implementation is to apply lean principles first, thereby eliminating the non-value-added process steps and creating flow. Six Sigma may then be employed to improve quality. Although a detailed explanation of the Six Sigma methodology and its implementation is beyond the scope of this book, what Six Sigma has to offer an organization is a topic worth exploring.

The concept of Six Sigma, including a statistical definition, a rationale, and a definition relating to the methodology, covers a lot of ground.

SIX SIGMA RATIONALE

The rationale behind Six Sigma indicates that the output of a process is a function of all the inputs. Stated mathematically, y (the output) is equal to a function of x (the inputs).

$$y = f(x)$$

There can be many inputs to a process. By minimizing the variation of these inputs, one can better predict the consistency of the output. W. Edwards Deming, the father of the Japanese post-war industrial recovery, coined the terms "special cause" and "common cause" to describe the two types of variation. Special-cause variation is the result of an arbitrary occurrence at some point in the process. Common-cause variation is the result of inconsistencies that are always present to some degree in every process. Six Sigma attempts to determine the inputs that are critical to quality (CTQ). Six Sigma incorporates many tools to aid in the identification of both types of variation. The eventual elimination or minimization of process variation with the intention of achieving a predetermined goal is the fundamental concept of Six Sigma.

SIX SIGMA STATISTICAL DEFINITION

Many books on the topic of Six Sigma discuss the application of the methodology, but fail to define the term from its statistical roots. To understand Six Sigma from a statistical perspective it is necessary to start with a fundamental question. What is a sigma? Sigma is the eighteenth letter of the Greek alphabet (Σ). It is used to denote the sum of a series of numbers. The lower-case sigma (σ) is used to denote standard deviation; it is this lower-case sigma referred to in the term Six Sigma. This information gives rise to the next question. What is a standard deviation? A standard deviation is roughly defined as the average distance from the average value of a set of numbers. Standard deviation is often defined as a measure of the spread; it indicates whether the data is clustered together or spread out. More formally, Six Sigma may be defined as plus or minus six standard deviations from the mean, or six average distances from the average value of a set of numbers.

Unless you possess a strong mathematical background, you may find this a bit confusing. Fortunately, a graphical representation makes this statistical concept much easier to understand. To begin, imagine a set of numbers generated by the output of a process. Consider the following set of numbers, which might represent the time, in minutes, required to conduct a certain test.

8, 10, 4, 9, 11, 6, 10, 12, 3, 5, 10, 2, 11, 7, 3, 8, 10, 8, 10, 9, 12, 11, 8, 10, 13, 15, 14, 13, 10, 14, 8, 17, 18, 7, 16, 9, 12, 10, 12, 11, 4, 5, 7, 10, 11, 7,12, 8, 9, 10, 13, 6, 14, 9, 15, 4, 6, 9, 13, 12, 9, 8, 10, 7, 12, 6, 8, 16, 9, 13, 12, 7, 10, 9, 14, 11, 9, 8, 13, 7, 11, 1, 14, 11, 15, 6, 10, 9, 11, 12, 19, 13, 11, 13, 11, 5, 18, 17, 2, 5, 12, 7, 16, 11, 9, 6, 10, 15, 8, 14, 16, 5, 13, 11, 3, 17, 12, 6, 10, 8, 15, 4, 7, 9, 14

If all these numbers were listed sequentially along a horizontal line with duplicate numbers stacked on top of each other, it would generate the histogram illustrated in Figure 9.1. This data produces what statisticians refer to as a normal distribution, what the rest of us call a bell-shaped curve. The mean, or average value, for this set of numbers is 10 (calculated by adding together all the numbers in the set and dividing the sum by how many numbers are in the set). The standard deviation, the average distance of these numbers from the mean, is 3.76 (calculated by finding the square root of the average squared distance of each value from the mean).

02	03	04	05	06	07	08	09	10	11	12	13	14	15	16	17	18
								10								
								10								
							09	10	11							
							09	10	11							
						08	09	10	11	12						
						08	09	10	11	12						
					07	08	09	10	11	12	13					
					07	08	09	10	11	12	13					
				06	07	08	09	10	11	12	13	14				
				06	07	08	09	10	11	12	13	14				
			05	06	07	08	09	10	11	12	13	14	15			
		04	05	06	07	08	09	10	11	12	13	14	15	16		
	03	04	05	06	07	08	09	10	11	12	13	14	15	16	17	
02	03	04	05	06	07	08	09	10	11	12	13	14	15	16	17	18

FIGURE 9.1   Histogram displaying a normal distribution.

For data with a normal distribution, the empirical rule relative to standard deviation implies that the area under the curve between one standard deviation below the mean and one standard deviation above the mean (1 sigma), contains 68.3 percent of the data. The area under the curve between two standard deviations below the mean and two standard deviations above the mean (2 sigma) contains 95.4 percent of the data. The area under the curve between three standard deviations below the mean and three standard deviations above the mean (3 sigma) contains 99.73 percent of the data. Therefore, three standard deviations or three sigma encompasses 99.73 percent of all the data. This is presented graphically in Figure 9.2.

Six standard deviations, or Six Sigma, encompasses 99.99966 percent of the data under the curve. After compensating for any drift (or shift), which occurs in any process, the 99.99966 percent translates to 3.4 defects per million opportunities (DPMO). Hence, the goal of a Six Sigma process is to have no more than 3.4 defects per million opportunities.

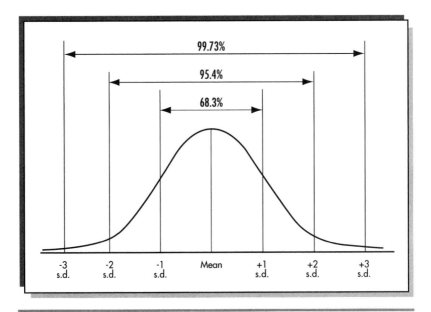

FIGURE 9.2   Percentage of area under the normally distributed curve for different sigma levels.

SIX SIGMA METHODOLOGY

The application of Six Sigma incorporates a methodology represented by the acronym DMAIC (pronounced duh-may-ick). DMAIC denotes the five phases of Six Sigma implementation: define, measure, analyze, improve, and control. Think of these five phases as follows:

- Define: What is the problem?
- Measure: How bad is the problem?
- Analyze: Under what circumstances does the problem occur?
- Improve: How can the problem be fixed?
- Control: How to ensure the problem stays fixed?

The DMAIC methodology provides a common process for teams to follow and incorporates numerous tools applicable to specific phases of implementation.

DEFINE

As with Lean, Six Sigma requires proper planning. Six Sigma employs a document called a project charter that is similar to the event planning worksheet. The same guidelines employed for the event planning worksheet outlined in Chapter 8: Conducting a Lean Event, may be applied to the project charter. There are, however, two sections in the project charter that do not appear on the event planning worksheet. These are business case and review timing.

The business case section asks why this project is important to the organization and how it relates to the strategic plan. A complete business case should also include the expected financial benefits afforded by the project and an explanation of how they were derived.

The review timing section is necessary to ensure the steady progression of the project. It is not uncommon for a Six Sigma project to continue for six months to a year before completion. Without the knowledge that a review is pending, the project could lose momentum. Even worse, it could stagnate completely and never reach completion.

MEASURE

In addition to the collection of data, the measure phase of the DMAIC process also requires confirming the accuracy of the measurement system and determining process capability.

Data collection requires critical thinking. It is important to ask the right question in regard to the data. Consider the set of numbers used to demonstrate a normal distribution. The usefulness of that data is nil unless we obtain additional information such as:

- What are the units? (minutes, days, pounds, milligrams, and so on)

- When was the data collected? (last week, last year, this morning)

- What method was employed to collect the data? (observation, computer generation, estimation)

- Over what period of time was the data collected? (seconds, years)

Depending on the process being measured, many more questions might be generated in relation to the data set. This questioning of the data set is critical to ensuring its validity and accuracy. The data collected during the measure phase is the baseline against which the improvements will be compared. The precision of these data is, therefore, critical to the success of the project.

Accuracy of the measurement system is equally vital to the project. If the measurement system is flawed in any way, the validity of the data is in question. Consequently, the analysis and subsequent improvements will be put into question. The old computer programming expression, "garbage-in, garbage-out," is an appropriate aphorism for the measurement phase of the DMAIC process. Six Sigma employs a measurement system analysis (MSA) to substantiate the measurement system. The measurement system analysis verifies the validity of the measurement device as well as the repeatability and reproducibility of the results.

Process capability, an important concept in Six Sigma, is defined as the ability of the process to remain within the spread of the specification limits. Two indices are used to designate process capability: *Cp* and *Cpk*. Cp defines the ability of the process to produce data that falls within the range created by the upper and lower specification limits. If Cp indicates that the process cannot produce data that is within the specification limits, the process must be improved or the specification limits changed. Cpk, on the other hand, identifies whether the process is centered within the specification limits and thereby acceptable. Centeredness (Cpk) can usually be attributed to a specific cause; adjustments can be made to center the process within the specification limits. The graphical representation of Cp and Cpk, illustrated in Figure 9.3, demonstrates the need for a process that is both capable and centered in order for the data to be acceptable.

Analyze

The analyze phase of the DMAIC process is where the real value of the methodology is demonstrated. Statistical analysis computes the probability and/or improbability that something will occur. The concepts and formulas associated with statistics originated from a desire to know and beat the odds associated with gambling. In Six Sigma, statistical analysis is used to demonstrate the impact of the process inputs on the process output. The data collected during the measure phase is analyzed to determine the probability of problems occurring in the process and to identify the cause of these problems. Extensive training is required to understand and apply the statistical tools available for use in the analysis phase. Pareto charts, hypothesis tests, correlation and regression analysis, and analysis of variance are only a smattering of the tools available. The causes identified during the analyze phase form the groundwork for the next phase in the process.

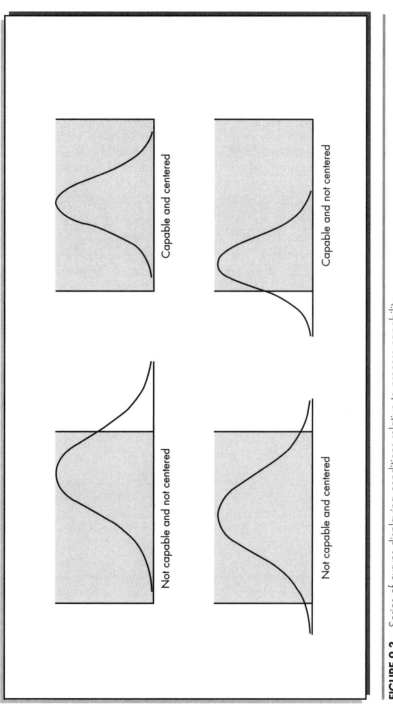

FIGURE 9.3   Series of curves displaying conditions relative to process capability.

IMPROVE

This phase involves developing, evaluating, refining, and implementing solutions for problems identified in the analyze stage. One of the more popular tools employed in the improve stage is design of experiment (DOE). Design of experiment allows the team to determine the effect of different proposed solutions on the process output. The result of a design of experiment often suggests employing one or more of the proposed solutions in varying degrees.

As with Lean, process improvements should be trialed and the results verified before implementation. Conducting improvements on a small scale will allow the team to adjust for any conditions that may have been overlooked.

CONTROL

The final phase of the DMAIC methodology is control. This phase involves documenting improvements and designing controls to ensure that process changes and improvements are adhered to and maintained. This phase assumes that the problem stays fixed and doesn't revert to the original state. In essence, it involves developing standard work. This is an essential step in any improvement initiative and is critical to maintaining the gains.

Six Sigma is a data-driven approach to quality improvement that employs statistical analysis to reduce or eliminate process variation and focuses on the customer's needs. It is much more than a scientific approach to quality improvement. Six Sigma also offers hospitals a methodology that complements the tools available in a lean transformation.

CONDUCTING A LEAN EVENT

A lean event is the dedication of a team of individuals whose sole purpose is to implement lean tools and concepts in a targeted area. From pre-event planning to the final presentation, no two lean events are ever the same. Each event proposes new challenges and new opportunities, and each event yields different results. The lean event is an exciting, action-packed, morale-boosting experience. Because lean requires bottom-up implementation, and because everyone in the organization has something to offer, everyone should have an opportunity to participate in at least one event. The combination of a team with experience and knowledge of the targeted area and a facilitator with the skill and understanding of lean tools and their application will produce extraordinary results.

Although no two events are alike, all events follow the five steps of standard work: evaluating the current situation, identifying areas of opportunity, modifying the existing process, substantiating and enumerating improvements, and implementing the new standard work (see Chapter 5: Standard Work).

Once an area has been targeted for a lean event, someone must be selected to lead it. A team must be organized and the scope, time frame, and objectives for the event must be established. Every event should culminate with a final team presentation. The final presentation allows all team members to take credit for what was accomplished during the event and shows management and anyone else who attends how much can be achieved. In addition, the final presentation is an opportunity for senior administrators to exhibit their commitment to the lean initiative by attending as many events as possible and praising the hard work and accomplishments of the team.

EVENT PLANNING

Almost every undertaking requires careful planning and a lean event is no exception. Careless planning will result in time wasted during the event. The event planning worksheet (see Figure 10.1) will assist in proper planning of the event. The following sections provide definitions for the information required on the form. Note that it is customary to provide a descriptive title for each event. Titles will help differentiate between events and help to create a team atmosphere.

Scope

The scope of the event defines where and on what the team will focus its efforts. It is important to be specific. In some cases it may be appropriate to indicate what is not included in the scope of the event as well as what is included. For example, if an event is targeted at reducing length of stay for pneumonia patients, the scope might include two specific diagnosis codes, DRG 89 and DRG 90. All other DRGs would be outside of the scope of the event.

It is important to be realistic when defining the scope of an event. A scope that is too aggressive will create frustration and stress for the team leader and the team's members. It is certainly acceptable to alter the scope during the first day or two of the event if it proves to be too aggressive or if some constraints or non-value-added activities are later identified as being outside of the original plan. Define the scope of a lean event as specifically as possible by first identifying the customer and considering value from that customer's point of view.

Dates

Although setting the dates for an event appears to be a relatively simple task, some considerations may be overlooked. One obvious consideration is the availability of the team leader, team members, the facilitator, and consultants. Other less obvious considerations must also be taken into account. Staffing shortages within the targeted area resulting from vacation leave, extended sick leave, or any other reason will complicate the attempt to conduct a lean event and will create havoc. Avoid seasons of excessively high patient volumes (such as flu season) if the targeted area is affected by increased volumes.

Event Objectives

Event objectives should incorporate the five components identified in the SMART acronym. Objectives must be specific, measurable, attainable, relevant, and time bound. Objectives are critical in the planning stage of the lean event. Without objectives, the team will wander aimlessly through the event and little, if anything, will be accomplished. The tendency is to be conservative when setting objectives, but lean events require a bias for getting things done. This will not happen if objectives are conservative. Use stretch objectives that will prompt action resulting from a sense of urgency and generate dramatic improvements. Objectives may be changed, but avoid the temptation to change for the sole purpose of having the results appear better

Event Planning Worksheet

Lean Hospitals
Bringing Lean to Healthcare

Scope:

Objectives:

Takt time:

Process information:

Dates:

Team leader:

Team members:

Facilitator:

Consultant:

Current situation and problems:

FIGURE 10.1 Event planning worksheet.

than they are. If it becomes evident that an objective is not realistic and cannot be accomplished as part of the event, create a plan to accomplish that objective after the event and add it to the continuous improvement to-do list (see Chapter 7).

To promote the use of kanbans and visual controls, include in the objectives the establishment of at least one of each.

Selecting a Team Leader

The appointment of an effective team leader is vital to the success of the lean event. The selected team leader must be committed to the success of the event and display buy-in to the lean strategy. A team leader who exhibits the slightest amount of even passive resistance to the change required for a lean transformation will yield results that fail to meet expectations. Do not assume that giving an individual the responsibility of leading an event will create buy-in; there is too much at risk.

An effective team leader must possess several important attributes including organization, leadership skills, commitment to the lean initiative, and a bias for getting things done. In addition, this individual should possess the ability to switch gears and focus on several objectives at the same time. It may appear that the team leader needs superhuman qualities; in fact, a surprising number of individuals in every organization are capable of filling this important role.

Organizing the Team

For a successful event to transpire, all team members must be willing to commit the time and energy necessary to make the event a success. No matter the amount of planning, no matter how dynamic the team leader or what level of facilitation, without an engaged, energetic, and committed team the event will surrender mediocre results at best. The individuals who make up the lean improvement team are entrusted with a great deal of responsibility, both to the hospital and to their fellow team members. Team members must understand the level of responsibility required. In addition to time and energy, each team member must be fully engaged in the process for the entire course of the event. Because so much must be accomplished during a lean event, individuals who need constant direction or who are unwilling to pull a fair share of the load are not suitable for inclusion on the team. An individual who possesses skills or knowledge essential to accomplishing the team's objectives but who is unable to commit the necessary time or level of engagement may be included as an ad-hoc team member who contributes his or her skills on an as-needed basis.

The size of the team will vary depending on the scope of the event. Although there is no rule of thumb for determining team size, a team should include a good composition of:

- *Skill* – An effective team needs individuals with the clinical and/or technical competence necessary to make changes to the value stream.

- *Cross-functional representation* – Most events will require crossing departmental boundaries. It is essential to have proper representation from these other areas in order to initiate any improvements for which they will be responsible.

- *Fresh eyes* – Sometimes we can't see the forest for the trees. Someone unfamiliar with the targeted area may add tremendous value to the improvement event because of a unique perspective.

PROCESS INFORMATION

Provide as much information as possible about the process. If a process map exists, attach it to the event planning worksheet. This will allow the team members to become familiar with the process beforehand. Do not use this information as part of the event. All information utilized during the event must be current, and will be obtained using the observation techniques described in Chapter 5.

CURRENT SITUATION AND PROBLEMS

A brief statement of the opportunities provided by this event is all that is necessary. Any available supporting data relative to opportunities should be attached to the event planning worksheet.

In addition to completing the event planning worksheet, you must communicate information regarding the event to all management and especially to those areas that may be directly or indirectly affected by any changes. Support services such as maintenance, information technology, environmental services, purchasing, finance, safety, and infection control must be notified of the event dates and the likelihood of need for their support.

Integral to adequate preparation is training. Although expertise in applying lean tools and concepts is something acquired only by participation in events, a rudimentary understanding of these tools and concepts and their application should be provided to all team members as part of the planning process. This training typically requires attendance at a three-day seminar on lean principles conducted by a consultant or by one of the organization's lean leaders. The training can be provided at any time, since a refresher is provided on the first day of any event.

The final step in the preparation process is to secure a room that will become the gathering place for the team, commonly referred to as the war room. Here the team will meet, brainstorm, work, and eat during the event. The room should be supplied with flip charts, markers, overhead projector, LCD projector, standard work forms, stopwatches, pens, pencils, rulers, tape, staples, work tables and chairs arranged in a manner conductive to the work taking place, and plenty of wall space to display charts, lists, and completed standard work forms. Comfort is not a concern; this is not a lounge but rather a place of action and excitement where improvement takes place.

The importance of proper planning can not be overstressed. It is essential to assure an event progress smoothly without hitches. Use the checklist provided in Figure 10.2 as a guide to assist in proper planning.

KICKING OFF THE LEAN EVENT

The lean event should be kicked off by a senior administrator, preferably the CEO or COO. This person should elaborate on the importance of the lean transformation to the organization and the responsibility entrusted to the team. He or she must illustrate the linkage to the strategic plan and emphasize the hospital's commitment to the team and their efforts.

Gemba is the next step in the event. Gemba is the Japanese word for the scene of the action. In this case it refers to where the process designated for improvement is performed. The entire team should visit the area with the team leader or area representative who can walk them through the process step-by-step. Don't attempt to simulate the gemba in the war room. A picture is worth a thousand words, but nothing replaces observing the process with your own two eyes.

Before starting the event by evaluating the current situation, the facilitator or consultant should conduct refresher training. This is not the time to conduct extensive workshop training. This training should focus on the use of standard work forms only, and should last no longer than two and a half hours. Refresher training for value stream mapping, kanban, visual controls, and other tools can be conducted during the event on an as-needed basis.

CONDUCTING THE EVENT

It's show time! The time has come to release team members to the targeted area and let them apply all they have learned. The first step is to document the current situation. Divide the team into groups of two and assign each group a specific task such as time observations. In this case, one person times the process step and the other records the data. Some tasks, such as creating a standard work sheet, will only require one person.

Lean Event Checklist

Complete the Event Planning Worksheet.

Schedule and conduct pre-event classroom training for team members as required (Overview and Standard Work at a minimum).

Obtain data relative to volumes and/or production requirements.

Obtain approvals or permits as required (some HR departments may require consent forms from employees being video taped).

Obtain visitor passes as required.

Issue a memo informing hospital management of the dates of the event.

Schedule a room to be used by the team for the entire event (War Room).

Inform team members of dates, start and end times, and location of the event.

Make arrangements for materials to be available in the war room (flip charts, projectors, pens, stopwatches, standard work forms, rulers, and so on).

Notify other departments of dates and their estimated support/involvement:

☐ Maintenance

☐ Environmental Services

☐ Quality

☐ Infection Control

☐ Safety

☐ Information Technology (IT)

☐ Purchasing

☐ Finance

☐ Human Resources

☐ Others _____

Calculate takt time   TT =

If food is being delivered, make arrangements for breaks and lunch.

Obtain floor plans of targeted areas.

Secure video cameras and viewing equipment.

Schedule an in-house facilitator or outside consultant to facilitate the event.

Schedule a representative from senior administration to help kick off the event.

Inform senior administration and all hospital directors of the date and time of the final presentation.

FIGURE 10.2   Lean event checklist.

Value stream maps, time observation forms, standard work sheets, takt time calculations, process maps, combination sheets, and percent load charts will quickly fill up the walls of the war room. Using this baseline information, the team will begin to identify opportunities and generate ideas to improve the process. This is an electrifying time and members will be energized and engaged. The level of exuberance will grow as new ideas are implemented and the team begins to see the process change for the better. Documentation of the current situation should be completed on the first day of the event; the team should already be generating ideas for improvement. Over the course of the remaining days the team will generate more ideas, begin to implement plans, and verify changes. During this time the team will also begin to implement lean tools: changeover improvements, mistake-proofing methods or devices, kanbans, and visual controls. The final day of the event is dedicated to tying up loose ends, developing the new standard work, and preparing for the final presentation.

At the end of each day the facilitator and team leader will meet to conduct a process check. They will review data, evaluate improvements, and verify that the team is on the right track. Sometimes adjustments must be made to redirect the team toward meeting the event objectives. In addition to ensuring that the team is on track, the facilitator and team leader evaluate participation of team members, the quality of the improvement ideas, the level of teamwork, and the spirit exhibited by the team. They then decide what action, if any, must be taken the following day to address concerns.

The last morning of the event the facilitator and team leader will work closely with the team members to verify and quantify the results. All improvements should be reflected in the new standard work for the process and documented using the applicable standard work forms. It is now time to prepare the final presentation.

THE FINAL PRESENTATION

As the event comes to a close, everyone in the organization will be eager to see what was accomplished. This is a real "feel good" time for the team, which has been engaged in non-stop activity directed toward improving the process. They will be exhausted and looking forward to the end of the event, but first they must be given an opportunity to expound what they have accomplished and take credit for their efforts. The final presentation is not executed by the team leader. Instead, every team member participates. This is important because it drives home the fact that this event was a team effort. Individuals who contributed great ideas during the event can now take credit for them. At the same time, the presentation demonstrates that it was the amalgamation of everyone's contribution that made the event a success. The final presentation should follow this sequence:

- *Team introduction* – Team member should introduce themselves to the audience and provide information about their jobs and departments.

- *Review objectives* – Show and explain the preliminary objectives that were set for the team. Do not talk about results at this point, only what the team was trying to accomplish.

- *Situation before the event* – Explain the situation that existed before the event. Present the standard work forms that were used to evaluate the original situation. Discuss with the audience the problems and opportunities the team was trying to address.

- *Accomplishments* – These are not the final results but rather the changes that were implemented during the event. Present the ideas generated by the team to eliminate non-value-added process steps. Identify the implementation of kanbans and visual controls that were incorporated, as well as mistake-proofing methods and changeover improvements.

- *Situation after the event* – Explain what the process looks like now. Use the new standard work forms that were generated to reflect the new process.

- *Results* – Show the team's preliminary objectives and the results obtained by the event. Don't be concerned if a 50 percent cycle time reduction was the objective and only 30 percent was achieved. Explain that preliminary objectives were stretch goals and quantify what the 30 percent reduction means in terms of time savings, dollar savings, and customer satisfaction.

- *Continuous improvement to-do list* – This will include a list of everything the team was not able to accomplish as part of the event. In spite of efforts to keep this list at a minimum, there will be occasions when it is just not possible to accomplish all improvements in the time allowed for the event. Explain what remains to be done, what results are expected, who is responsible, and when the final improvements will be completed.

- *Questions and answers* – There will be many questions. Although questions should normally be answered by the team member assigned to a particular task, this is not a hard and fast rule. The objective is to demonstrate everyone's level of involvement in the event, so the team leader should be prepared to come to the aide of a team member who may have little or no experience speaking in front of a group.

It may be necessary to conduct several final presentations to ensure that everyone has the opportunity to see and hear the results of the event. This is vital to the success of the lean transformation. Communicating the successes and allowing other staff members to see and hear that lean really works will go a long way toward creating the culture change required for the lean transformation.

IV ADMIXTURE LEAN EVENT
YALE-NEW HAVEN HOSPITAL

Yale-New Haven Hospital (YNHH) is one of the oldest hospitals in the nation. Located in New Haven, it is Connecticut's first and the nation's fourth voluntary hospital. A not-for-profit organization, it is the primary teaching hospital for Yale University School of Medicine. It is a 944-bed facility that includes Yale-New Haven Children's Hospital and Yale-New Haven Psychiatric Hospital. The July 18th, 2005 issue of U.S. News & World Report ranked YNHH among the nation's top hospitals for the fourteenth consecutive year and among the nation's top 100 hospitals in 10 of the 17 specialties evaluated. Being on the cutting edge of technology and consistently looking for new and innovative improvement methods has kept YNHH among America's best hospitals and has earned it the recognition and reputation it justly deserves.

YNHH recognizes the potential for lean in healthcare and has already begun lean implementation in its organization. An early lean event conducted in the Yale-New Haven Hospital Pharmacy targeted the Intravenous (IV) Admixture service. Team members attended a two-day lean training session one month prior to the event. The following is an overview of the five-day lean event and an example of real-life application of lean principles.

PHARMACY DEPARTMENT –
IV ADMIXTURE LEAN EVENT

The IV Admixture service operates twenty-four hours a day, seven days a week, three hundred and sixty-five days a year in order to meet the demands of all adult and pediatric IV medication orders. This high-volume service, which is experiencing significant growth, fills and delivers more than 650 orders daily.

THE TEAM

The team included seven pharmacists, one pharmacy resident, two pharmacy compounding technicians, and one nurse practitioner (See Figures 11.6a, 11.6b, 11.6c, and 11.6d).

Team Leader: Lorraine A. Lee, R.Ph.
Manager, Medication Safety and Regulatory Compliance
Director, Pharmacy Practice Residency

Co-Leader: Sandra McKelvie Bacon, A.P.R.N.
Performance Improvement Coordinator

Team Members: Edward Silva, Pharm.D.
Pharmacy Operations Specialist

Eric Cabie, M.B.A., R.Ph.
Pharmacy Operations Specialist

Norbert Robinson, R.Ph.
Manager, Pharmacy Operations

Michelle Benish, Pharm.D.
Clinical Coordinator, Education and Training

Phuong Sander, Pharm.D.
Pediatric Clinical Pharmacist

Tram Phan, Pharm.D.
Clinical Pharmacist

Shawn Thomas
Pharmacy Technician II

Sheila Munroe
Pharmacy Technician III

Maribeth Pauli, Pharm.D.
Pharmacy Practice Resident

THE PROBLEM STATEMENT

The scope of the event focused on a complex process that began at the time an order was entered into the system by the person prescribing the medication and ended when the medication left the Pharmacy for delivery to the unit. Regulatory guidelines developed by U.S. Pharmacopoeia (USP797) to govern pharmacies that prepare "compounded sterile preparations" (CSP) made the process somewhat cumbersome and did not support efficient production flow. As a result, products were manufactured in batches and in anticipation of patient needs, "just in case." The area was relatively small and congested, and there were numerous interruptions.

In addition to the apparent inefficiencies in the process, the quantity of returned and unused product was extremely high. Compounding this problem, expiration dates made it necessary to discard most of the IV drip orders returned to the Pharmacy. Product delivery methods were unreliable. A compounded medication sometimes waited in the pass-through refrigerator for more than an hour before someone on the receiving side became aware that it was ready to be queued in the pneumatic tube system for delivery. Reorders were common. Most of them occurred when clinicians on the units did not receive the original order quickly enough. In some observed cases, a product waited for delivery in the pass-through refrigerator while a compounding technician manufactured the same product as a reorder.

EVALUATE THE CURRENT SITUATION

The first step of the event was to evaluate the current situation. This began with a gemba (a visit to the location where the process is performed). The team was escorted to the sterile production area where the team leader walked everyone through the process step-by-step.

After a prescribed order is entered electronically into the database and verified by a pharmacist, a label is printed in the IV Admixture room with the medication order. The compounding technician uses standard recipe cards to set up the order by obtaining the diluents, drugs, and supplies. A manufacturing label is generated employing the standard recipe cards for expiration dates. The same or another compounding technician then prepares the medication using aseptic techniques in a laminar flow hood. At that point, all vials and ampoules used in preparation, syringes (with plunger pulled back indicating volume of ingredient used), calculation sheets, and the final labeled product are placed in a tray for verification by the pharmacist. The pharmacist validates the accuracy of each active ingredient and the volume used compared to the original order. In addition, the pharmacist independently performs all calculations and checks them against the calculations of the compounding technician. The finished product is then placed in queue for the appropriate delivery mechanism.

The area was a labyrinth of activity, with everyone working feverishly. Orders were being set up and placed in queue (see Figure 11.1a). Scheduled orders, new orders, and reorders were spewing from the label printer. Wire racks covered with defrosting product were moved to wherever there was room (Figure 11.1b). Pharmacists and technicians moved hurriedly about the room searching for supplies, diluents, and drugs. Oftentimes staff members were required to leave the area to obtain what was needed. This required the removal and disposal of shoe covers and bouffant and the donning of new ones prior to reentry (see Figure 11.1c).

The gemba was an eye-opening look at the existing situation; it started team members on the path to an improved process.

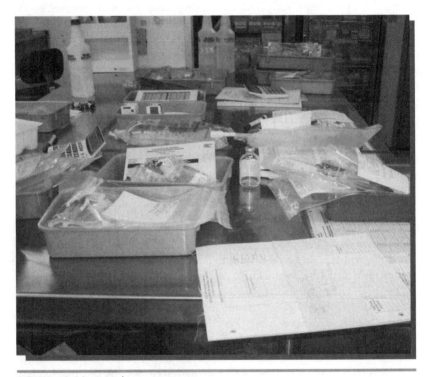

FIGURE 11.1A Work in process.

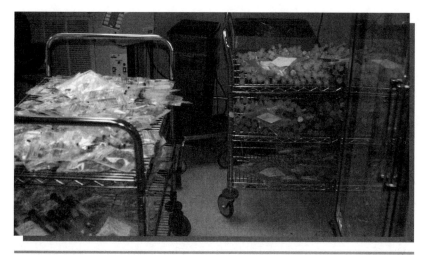

FIGURE 11.1B   Product defrosting on carts.

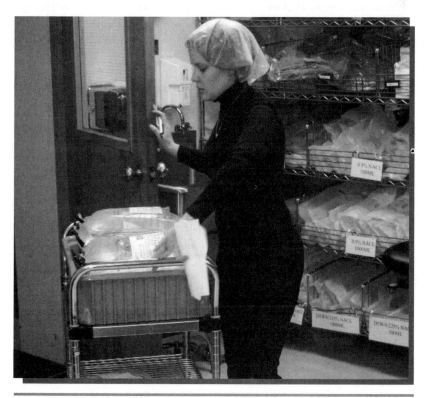

FIGURE 11.1C   Molly Billstein, Pharm.D., MICU Clinical Pharmacist, returning to area with diluents.

Calculate Takt Time

The next step was to determine customer demand and to evaluate the service's ability to meet that demand. This was accomplished by calculating the takt time and using timed observations to determine the cycle times for compounding medications.

The wide variety of products, and the understanding that each order was patient specific, made it necessary to group products into categories or families. After some discussion, four categories were identified and the total daily volume determined for each.

- Type A   Pre-made medications: 36% – 243 units

- Type B   Simple, Patient Specific: 40% – 264 units

- Type C   Moderate, Patient Specific: 23% – 153 units

- Type D   Complicated medications: 1% – 6 units

Since the service operates twenty-four hours a day with each 8-hour shift having two 15-minute breaks, the daily time available is 1350 minutes. This number was used to calculate Takt time:

- Type A   1350 / 243 = 5.56 minutes per unit

- Type B   1350 / 264 = 5.11 minutes per unit

- Type C   1350 / 153 = 8.82 minutes per unit

- Type D   1350 / 6 = 225 minutes per unit

These takt times appeared to be long, considering the level of activity witnessed in the IV Admixture room. Further discussion with the team revealed that more than 65 percent of the medication orders required for the day were filled in a six-and–a-half hour timeframe between 7:00 a.m. and 1:30 p.m. It became obvious that it would be necessary to calculate three takt times for each category. Based on customer demand, the takt time for the 7:00 a.m. to 1:30 p.m. timeframe was calculated as follows (allowing for three 15-minute breaks):

- Type A   *345 / 160 = 2.16 minutes per unit*

- Type B   *345 / 147 = 2.35 minutes per unit*

- Type C   *345 / 125 = 2.76 minutes per unit*

- Type D   *345 / 3 = 115 minutes per unit*

Another piece of information critical to the takt time calculation was the fact that not all products involved compounding. Only 20 percent of Type B, 40 percent of Type C, and 100 percent of Type D orders required compounding. The remaining orders involved the bagging and tagging of pre-made or purchased products and could be categorized with Type A orders. The final takt time calculations are shown in Table 11.1. These numbers included reorders that, if reduced or eliminated, would result in an increase in the takt times.

Once the takt times were calculated, the team was ready to begin documenting the current situation. This involved going to the sterile production area, conducting time observations, and completing the other standard work forms. Before releasing the team, refresher training was conducted on the use of the standard work forms including the standard work sheet (Figure 5.3), time observation sheet (Figure 5.6), combination sheet (Figure 5.8), and the percent loading chart (Figure 5.11). The team members were then given assignments to observe and document the different processes and products.

The processes to be documented included the setting up of orders, the compounding of products, the verification of orders, and the delivery of the four different product categories. Observations were difficult to obtain because of the lack of a standardized work sequence and the constant interruptions experienced by the staff. Although the IV Admixture staff members worked earnestly to complete the day's orders and each person did whatever was necessary to complete the tasks at hand, the sequence in which they performed their duties was often random or disrupted for various reasons. The inability to obtain time observations created the need to have the staff follow sequential process steps.

TABLE 11.1   Takt time calculations.

Product	7:00 am – 1:30 pm **345 minutes**	1:30 – 11:30 pm **525 minutes**	11:30 pm – 7:00 am **390 minutes**
Type A	345/353 = 59 sec.	525/98 = 5.36 min.	390/95 = 4.1 min.
Type B	345/29 = 11.9 min.	525/10 = 52.5 min.	390/13 = 30.0 min.
Type C	345/50 = 5.75 min.	525/8 = 65.6 min.	390/4 = 97.5 min.
Type D	345/3 = 115 min.	525/3 = 175 min.	N/A

In order to get a better understanding of the specific process steps, standard work sheets were reviewed. Rather than drawing the room layout on each sheet, a floor plan was used as the standard work sheet. The set-up process illustrated on the standard work sheet in Figure 11.2 involved pulling a recipe card, obtaining the drugs and diluents, and printing a manufacturing label. Surprisingly, these few tasks involved eighteen steps, most of them non-value-added, including but not limited to searching, clarifying, and restocking supplies that had run out.

Because of all the non-value-added activity associated with the process steps, it was easy for the staff members to deviate from any sequence. It was, therefore, necessary to instruct the staff members being observed to follow a specific sequence of tasks for each order. In the case of set-up, this meant: pull the recipe card, obtain the drug, obtain the diluents, and print the label. Even after establishing a process sequence, it was nearly impossible to obtain an uninterrupted observation of all four process steps. Asking staff to follow the defined process sequence made it possible to document the source of the non-value-added activity associated with the task. These comments provided the basis on which to focus the improvement efforts. The same was true for the manufacturing process, which was further complicated by the compounding technician's need to leave the area of the laminar flow hood to obtain an item. Each time this happened, the technician was required to put on a clean gown and gloves before returning to the sterile work area of the laminar flow hood.

Time observations were completed and cycle times were established for each product group. The cycle times were then multiplied by product quantities to determine whether cycle times (the rate at which the work is done) were able to meet demand (the rate at which work needs to be done). The percent loading chart for filling orders in the 7:00 a.m. to 1:30 p.m. time frame is shown in Figure 11.3. Because of the various product categories and assorted takt times, the available time of 345 minutes was used as a target indicator (390 minutes minus three 15-minute breaks). The time necessary for all four staff members to complete their tasks exceeded the target. This was confirmed by the fact that many of the adult and pediatric IV Drip orders were not ready for delivery at 1:30 p.m. These had to be included in a subsequent delivery that began at 4:30 p.m. In order to complete all orders for delivery by 1:30 p.m., it would be necessary to reduce the overall cycle time by more than 4 hours.

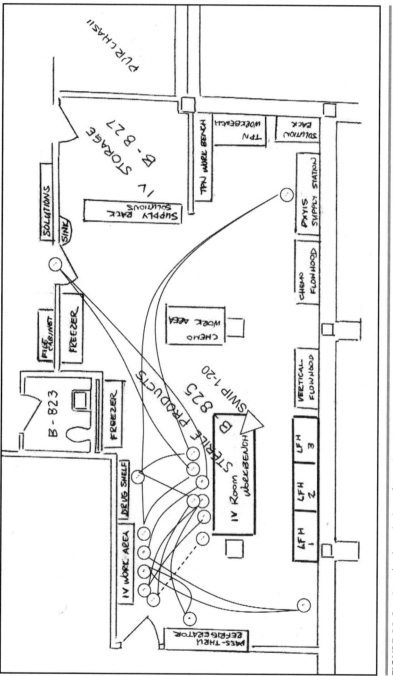

FIGURE 11.2   Standard work sheet for order setup.

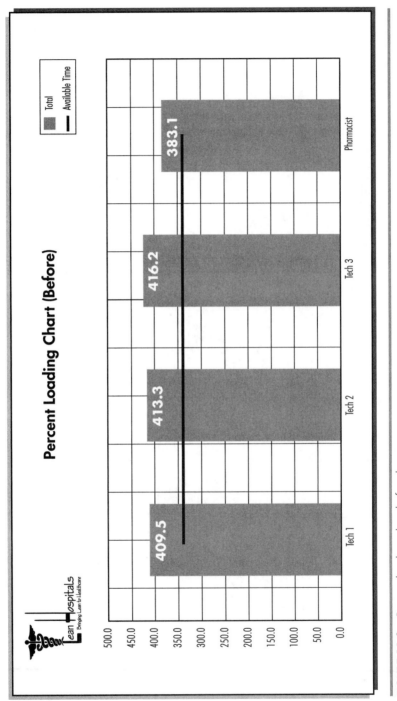

FIGURE 11.3 Percent loading chart before lean.

IDENTIFY AREAS OF OPPORTUNITY

The most commonly documented cause of disruption to flow was related to not having the drugs, diluents, or supplies readily available for use. In one case, it was observed that the entire content of a bin of diluents was needed for a single order; subsequent orders required that someone leave the room to obtain additional diluents and replenish the room supply. In most cases, the non-value-added work associated with a specific task was nearly equal to the value-added work. If the staff member had to leave the IV Admixture room to replenish the room stock, the non-value-added portion of the task time could more than triple. It became obvious early on that the first improvement activity would be to organize the work area (5S) and establish par levels for drugs, diluents, and supplies. It would also be necessary to set up kanbans to ensure that par levels were maintained and supplies replenished when necessary.

Par levels were established by determining usage history, identifying the response time for obtaining items from in-house or outside suppliers, and establishing buffers. Buffers were established based on past experience relative to stock outs, fluctuations in demand, and erratic delivery cycles. The par level was established using this formula:

$$\text{Par Level} \;=\; \text{Daily Usage} \;\times\; \frac{\text{Response Time}}{\text{Order Size}} \;\times\; \text{Buffer}$$

For example: daily usage of a particular drug is 50 vials, it takes the supplier two days to refill an order, the order size is 100 vials, and past experience suggests a buffer of 20%. The par level would be calculated as follows:

$$50 \text{ vials} \;\times\; \frac{2 \text{ days}}{100 \text{ vials/order}} \;\times\; 1.2 \;=\; 1.2 \text{ orders}$$

Based on this calculation, a par level of 120 vials is necessary (1.2 orders multiplied by 100 vials per order).

In order to ensure that items are replenished as needed, it was necessary to establish kanbans. Kanban cards were implemented for products manufactured in the IV Admixture room and stored in the refrigerator. The kanban card signaled the need for replenishment and products were manufactured at times other than peak order fill time, mainly on the evening shift. The percent load chart created for the evening shift established that there was available time on evenings to accomplish this and other tasks. The team elected to use the double-bin method for drugs, diluents, and supplies, counting on the empty bin to act as the kanban and signal the need for replenishment (see Figure 3.6).

MODIFY THE EXISTING PROCESS

The next step was to establish standard work based on the value-added times recorded during time observations. The value-added time required to manufacture a medication order was 103 seconds for a Type B product and 375 seconds for a Type C product. Type D products required long wait times during compounding, but the value-added portion was similar to a Type C product. The value-added portion of set up required 56 seconds. Based on this information, it was obvious that one compounding technician could be setting up orders while two other technicians manufactured orders. This freed the pharmacist to focus on verifying orders rather than assisting with setting up orders. With par levels established and kanbans in place, it became unnecessary for the technicians or pharmacist to fetch supplies due to stock-outs of the room's supply.

To facilitate the standard work, the IV room workbench was divided into three sections using colored tape. The three sections were designated work in process, completed set-ups, and compounded medications ready for verification (see Figure 11.4). The set-up technician, in addition to setting up orders, was also responsible for preparing half of the pre-made product for delivery (all Type A and some Type B and C). Preparation of pre-made product involved placing the pre-made product in a bag and securing a label; this took 73 seconds. Standard work in process was two orders in process and four orders set up and ready. The set-up trays were color coded to indicate priority. Scheduled orders used a green tray, new orders or reorders used a blue tray, and stat orders used a red tray. Set-ups were pulled by the compounding technicians working at the laminar flow hoods. The compounding technician assigned to the set-up sequence would set up the next order only when one of the compounding technicians working at the laminar flow hood moved a completed order to the verification section and pulled the next order from the completed set-ups. The resulting pull system ensured that orders were not batched, reducing the possibility for error, maintaining established priorities, and reinforcing proper flow. The pharmacist's primary function became the verification of orders. Implementing standard work meant that the only time the pharmacist was required to deviate from verifying orders was to set up a stat order and move it to the front of the standard work-in-process queue, indicating priority by using a red tray (a visual signal). The percent loading chart created after implementing the new standard work is shown in Figure 11.5. By following the new standard work, all orders were filled, verified, and ready for the 1:30 delivery run.

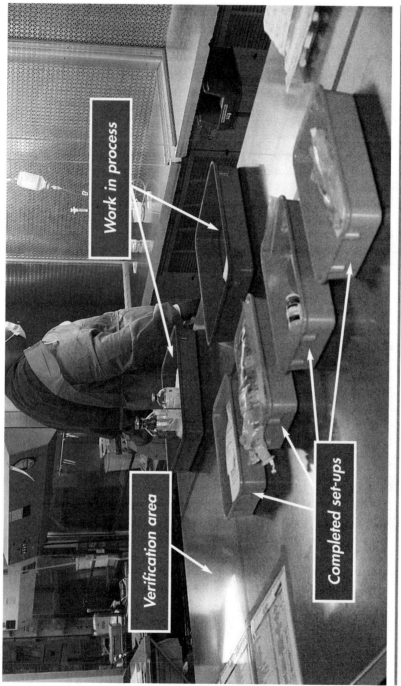

Work in process

Verification area

Completed set-ups

FIGURE 11.4 Example of established standard work.

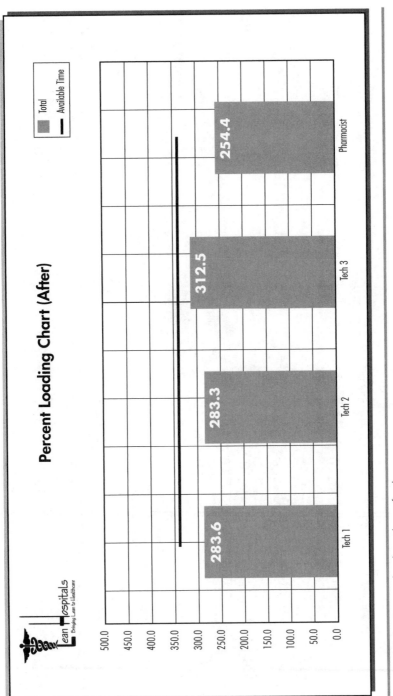

FIGURE 11.5 Percent loading chart after lean.

Other improvements included moving the order label printer to the top of the workbench. In its former location under the workbench, orders could go unnoticed for relatively long periods of time (see Figure 11.6e); this affected the turnaround time. Moving the printer to the top of the workbench adjacent to the pharmacist's computer terminal (see Figure 11.6f) allowed it to serve as a visual signal that an order was being received. The staff was now able to begin processing an order as soon as the label printed, and this simple change reduced turnaround time.

The IV syringe usage report, which normally printed at 6:30 a.m., told the staff which product needed to be pulled from the freezer, defrosted, labeled, and stored for usage during the day. A pharmacy technician scheduled to arrive at 6:30 a.m. each day removed items from the freezer and laid them out on wire racks for defrosting (see Figure 11.1b). The time required to defrost product was approximately two hours. Another technician was required to label and put away the product starting at about 8:30 a.m. Because this coincided with peak order-fill time, it created a disruption to flow. In addition, product was often not fully defrosted and ready for use when it was needed, causing additional delays. In order to remedy this condition, the IV syringe usage report was scheduled to print again at 7:00 p.m. This additional report provided information to the evening shift, prompting them to remove the syringes from the freezer at 7:00 p.m., lay them out for defrosting, label them, and put them away at 9:00 p.m. This not only did away with the defrosting carts cluttering the area (see Figure 11.1b), but also allowed the morning staff to maintain the standard work sequence without disruption. It eliminated the waiting associated with defrosting product during the peak order fill time of 7:00 a.m. to 1:30 p.m

A requisition was submitted to the maintenance department to install a pass-through window and andon light next to the pharmacist's computer terminal. This allows the pharmacists to deliver completed orders to the pneumatic tube stations, located on the opposite side of the wall, without having to take off shoe covers and bouffant and put on new ones prior to returning to the IV Admixture room. The andon light provides a visual signal that alerts the staff outside of the IV Admixture room that a medication order is ready for delivery and ready to be queued in the pneumatic tube system.

The pass-through window ensures that orders do not sit in the pass-through refrigerator for long periods of time before being queued in the pneumatic tube system. Accordingly, orders reach the unit as quickly as possible, resulting in a significant decrease in both turnaround time and reorders.

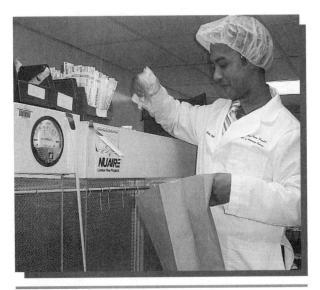

FIGURE 11.6A Eric Cabie, M.B.A., R.Ph., Pharmacy Operations Specialist, organizing supplies.

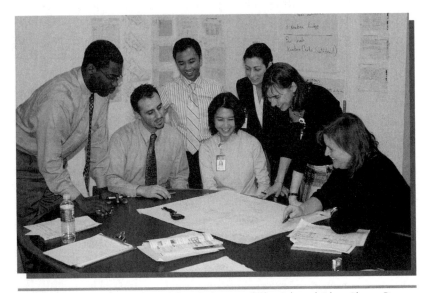

FIGURE 11.6B Left to right; Norbert Robinson, R.Ph., Edward Silva, Pharm.D., Eric Cabie, M.B.A., R.Ph., Phuong Sander, Pharm.D., Sandra McKelvie Bacon, A.P.R.N., Lorraine A. Lee, R.Ph., Michelle Benish, Pharm.D., reviewing the future time line.

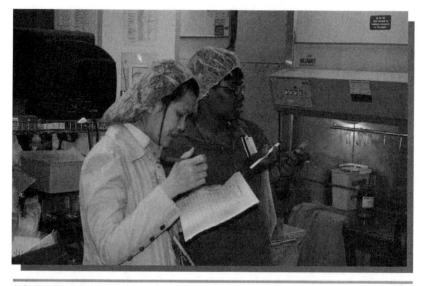

FIGURE 11.6C   Tram Phan, Pharm.D. and Sheila Munroe doing time observations.

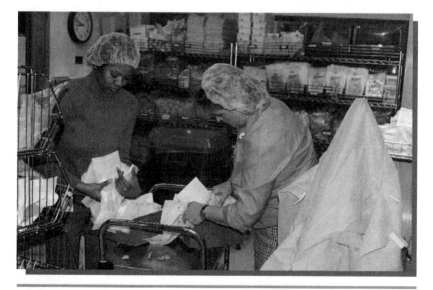

FIGURE 11.6D   Shawn Thomas and Michelle Benish, Pharm.D., sorting supplies.

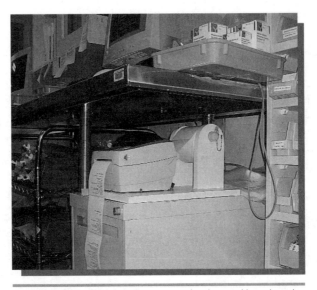

FIGURE 11.6E The label printer under the workbench with printed orders.

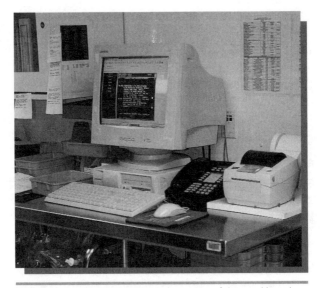

FIGURE 11.6F The label printer on top of the workbench next to the pharmacist's terminal.

A current state time line was drawn showing staffing levels, order print times, delivery times for adult and pediatric intermittent orders, and adult and pediatric IV drip orders over a twenty-four hour period. The time line identified that compounded medication orders could sit in the IV Admixture room, awaiting delivery, for up to nine hours. It also illustrated that many orders were manufactured prior to peak new-order time when physicians made their rounds and changed or discontinued medications. This resulted in compounded medications that were no longer required or now inappropriate due to changes in dosage. Rescheduling shift start and end times, delivery times, and the times the various reports printed reduced from nine hours to three and a half hours the maximum amount of time that a scheduled order could wait for delivery. Printing pediatric IV drip orders after the peak new-order entry time, at 1:00 p.m. instead of 8:00 a.m., resulted in fewer changed or discontinued orders being manufactured.

Most of the IV drip orders returned to the pharmacy were the result of orders discontinued or orders sent as reorders. In some cases, the pharmacy was not notified that an IV drip rate had been changed thereby changing the daily demand. The team estimated that the pharmacist spent at least one hour a day on the telephone with the various units, attempting to confirm whether or not IV drip orders were still active and verifying the current drip rate. The team recommended that the unit's clinical pharmacist notify the IV Admixture room of any discontinued medications or rate changes on a daily basis. This would appreciably reduce the manufacture of discontinued medications.

Yet another reason for reorders was the inability of the clinicians on the units to find the delivered medications due to multiple delivery and storage locations. By standardizing the delivery and storage locations for IV medications and notifying the unit staff members of these locations, reorders were reduced even further.

During observations it became apparent that the technicians spent too much time looking for the specific recipe cards needed for an order. This non-value-added searching was the result of the cards not being returned to their proper alphabetical location in card file. To facilitate returning recipe cards to their proper locations, each card was numbered. New cards were were assigned a letter in addition to the number associated with its location in the file. For example, a card to be filed between card 7 and card 8 was labeled 7A. To facilitate proper re-filing of the recipe cards, a place holder was inserted whenever a recipe card was removed. Another problem had to do with recipe cards that were not updated regularly. Information on the cards did not always agree with information in the computer or in the standard. Clarifying and verifying information on the recipe cards resulted in additional delays for the pharmacist, who had to stop what he or she was doing to cross check the various information sources for the technician. Standard work was set in place making it the responsibility of the pharmacy operations specialists to change the information in the pharmacy database and print, laminate, and file new recipe cards whenever a new standard was issued.

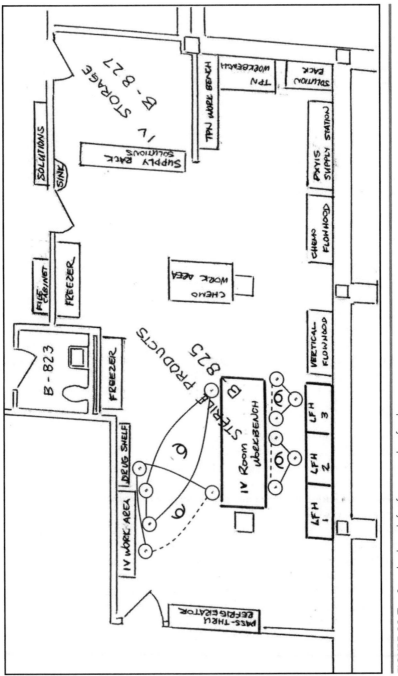

FIGURE 11.7 Standard work for four people after lean.

SUBSTANTIATE AND ENUMERATE IMPROVEMENTS

Because the par levels and kanbans were not yet in place by the last day of the event, it was necessary to simulate the condition by ensuring that all items were fully stocked prior to implementing the standard work. Flow was established using the new standard work sequence illustrated on the standard work sheet in Figure 11.7. The standard work sheet shows the work sequence and process sequence for four people: a set-up technician, two compounding technicians, and a pharmacist.

The four-person sequence creates a steady flow of production from setting up the order through to delivery via the pass-through window or other delivery mechanism. Based on the value-added cycle times, the set-up technician has time available to label and package pre-made Type A and some Type B and Type C orders and still maintain the four-order setup that was the standard work in process. The pharmacist could now focus his or her attention on the verification of orders, thereby reducing the likelihood of errors. The process was significantly less hectic and more structured after standard work implementation.

By eliminating the non-value-added process steps associated with the set up of orders, set-up times were reduced to less than a minute. This translated to an 80 percent reduction in the cycle time required for order set up. This reduction applied to approximately 80 percent of the orders. Orders of medications from the Pyxis system required an additional 30 to 60 seconds. The team recommended that the Pyxis system be relocated closer to the IV room workbench by switching its location with that of the freezer.

Cycle-time reductions were also achieved relative to compounding medications. Cycle times went from 176 seconds to 103 seconds for Type B products, a 41 percent cycle-time reduction, and from 548 seconds to 375 seconds for Type C products, a 32 percent cycle-time reduction.

Identifying discontinued orders, manufacturing orders after peak new-order times, and shortening turnaround times is expected to result in a 50 percent drop in the amount of discarded product and the number of reorders. Actual numbers were not available at the time of this writing.

IMPLEMENT STANDARD WORK

The final and most difficult phase of any lean event is getting the staff to follow the new standard work. Many of the changes necessary to incorporate flow are counterintuitive. The tendency is to return to the status quo and what "feels" right. Only by regularly monitoring that the IV Admixture room staff is following the newly established standard work will the benefits be fully realized. This is the responsibility of management. This is a difficult task but, over time, the new standard work will become the accepted process and will begin to "feel" right.

TABLE 11.2 Quantified results.

	Before	**After**	**% Improvement**
Set-up	285 seconds	56 seconds	80%
Compounding Type B	176 seconds	103 seconds	41%
Compounding Type C	548 seconds	375 seconds	32%
Verification	59 seconds	35 seconds	41%
Delivery to tube system	107 minutes	15 seconds	99.7%
* Total for Type B	554 seconds	205 seconds	63%
* Total for Type C	753 seconds	331 seconds	56%
* Does not include time for delivery to pneumatic tube system			

In order to continue moving forward, the management and staff of the IV Admixture service need to always be attentive to anything that disrupts flow. They must take immediate action to eliminate the cause of any deviation from standard work. This awareness of non-value-added tasks and the empowerment to take action will lead to the development of a lean mentality. For example, if a medication set up requires leaving the room to obtain a drug, it is necessary to determine why the drug was not available and what must be done to make it available in the future.

SUMMARY

The objectives for this event were to decrease turnaround time for new medication orders, decrease waste of returned and unused product, decrease the number of reorders, improve efficiency, and maintain medication safety.

By establishing par levels and implementing kanbans for drugs, diluents, and supplies, non-value-added process steps were reduced or eliminated, making the process more efficient and reducing turnaround time (see Table 11.2).

Timely information about discontinued orders, standardized delivery locations, pediatric IV drip orders printed after the peak new-order time, and decreased turnaround and delivery times for IV medications will contribute to the reduction of IV Admixture reorders. Over time, this will translate into decreased waste of returned and unused product.

Finally, allowing the pharmacist to focus on the verification of orders and the accuracy of the compounded product will contribute to maintaining the level of medication safety necessary for the IV Admixture service.

Reprinted with permission from Yale-New Haven Hospital.

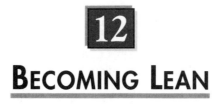

BECOMING LEAN

The preceding chapters have provided all the information any hospital administrator needs to begin a lean transformation This is a major undertaking that requires sincere commitment, unwavering patience, and considerable time. The end results, however, make it well worth the effort. Make no mistake about the level of commitment required for this undertaking. Many manufacturing companies have taken on this venture and failed miserably because of a lack of commitment. The old methods of doing business were too deeply ingrained in the culture of the company, and the level of commitment too feeble to create the change. For the Japanese it was a matter of survival, a need to reestablish their country as well as their business in the global economy. This is a level of dedication foreign to many American manufacturing companies. Nonetheless, many have risen the occasion and turned their businesses around, creating lean enterprises that would rival Toyota. Becoming a lean hospital is not a pipe dream; it is a very real, very achievable aspiration, but it must be done right.

SERVICE AND PRODUCT GROUPS

In order to create flow it is necessary to first identify all the service and product groups within the hospital. A service or product group may be defined as any group of services or products required by the patient/customer. There may be many services or products within a group. The surgical services group, for example, may include general surgery, orthopedic surgery, cardiac surgery, neurosurgery, and vascular surgery. Map the value stream for each group, not for each service. Concentrate on one service or product group at a time. Otherwise, the map will encompass everything that takes place in the hospital. For example, if a service group includes the need for an x-ray, do not map the process through the x-ray department. Because the x-ray department services many other departments as well as providing outpatient services, mapping the value stream through x-ray would complicate the map without adding value. Simply show x-ray as a process step within the value stream. Be aware that many times the value stream itself will overlap other value streams. This is expected and must be dealt with.

Within each product or service group the goal is to create flow for patients and products. Establishing standard work, making the process user-friendly, and providing unobstructed throughput are the key concepts of lean transformation. User-friendly means providing, for both patient and staff, what is needed, when it's needed, in the quantity needed, on time, every time, twenty four hours a day, seven days a week, three hundred and sixty five days a year. This requires the establishment of kanbans and and the implementation of visual controls because it's impossible to maintain standard work if supplies are not readily available, if people must seek clarification or verification, if equipment is not in working order, or if workarounds or stop-gap measures are in place.

A LEAN MENTALITY

To become a lean hospital requires that management first create a new culture, one where change is the only constant. It requires a paradigm shift away from one way of thinking to another. A shift away from accepting things the way they are, from believing that mistakes are an inevitable consequence of the complexity of the care delivery process. A shift toward a culture that has no tolerance for non-value-added process steps, one that knows that mistakes can be prevented and their impact mitigated. In this culture the patient/customer defines value and pulls that value from the process.

Everyone in the organization must develop a heightened awareness of value and the ability to identify and eliminate non-value-added tasks. This level of awareness can best be illustrated by the following story.

In 1863, a fifteen-year-old boy walked into the offices of the Grand Trunk Railroad Company in Ontario, Canada in response to an advertisement he had seen for a job as a telegraph operator. When he entered the building, a long line of men, all older than he, were waiting to apply for the job. The line stretched from the manager's office out to the hallway, down the length of the hall, and down the stairs into the lobby. Undaunted, the young man stood at the end of this very long line and watched the hustle and bustle of the workers. People were running around with important messages that had just been received over the telegraph lines. Managers were barking orders, workers were calling out to each other. . . . In the background was the ever-present telegraph-office sound, the dots and dashes of hundreds of Morse code messages being transmitted and received. Suddenly this boy stepped away from the line, walked up the stairs, down the hallway, and through the office area. He hesitated only slightly in front of the manager's office, but then opened the office door and walked in. Closing the door behind him this young boy declared, "I want this job." The manager, a burly man, stepped out from behind his desk, opened the office door, and announced to the waiting men that they could all go home. He had found the man he was looking for. One might think it was sheer boldness that allowed this young boy to land a highly sought after job, but that was not the case. That morning, among all the messages being transmitted and received in the company's office, one Morse code message was repeated over and over. Every person standing in that line heard it. The message simply said, "If you want this job, come into my office and tell me you want it." Only the young boy possessed the heightened awareness necessary to discern that message from all the others being transmitted that day and take appropriate action. His name was Thomas Alva Edison, very likely the most successful inventor in recorded history. He eventually held 1,093 patents that earned him the title of "the Wizard of Menlo Park."

The awareness young Thomas Edison exhibited by segregating that single message from all the others is analogous to the level of awareness sought in a lean organization. Employees must be able to isolate those operations that do not add value from all the other action occurring in the workplace. When this level of awareness is achieved, the organization has developed a lean mentality. This is not the end of the lean transformation; it is the beginning of the end of the outdated care delivery process. It is the beginning of a new era for the organization, an era in which patients receive high-quality care and the hospital prospers

A NEVER-ENDING JOURNEY

The pursuit of perfection knows no end. The leaders of a lean hospital must never become complacent with the progress of their lean transformation. Given the opportunity, complacency will rob the organization of all it has accomplished, slowly, mercilessly, and completely. This is not to say that the journey will not become easier with experience, only that it is necessary to remain constantly vigilant in the pursuit of perfection.

The same level of leadership required to launch the lean initiative is required to maintain it. An organization's leaders must be visible, they must be engaged, and they must keep lean principles in the forefront of organizational pursuits. Growth is a typical outcome of a lean transformation. As a result of the improved efficiency of hospital processes, increased revenues, and freed-up resources, expansion of services becomes an obvious course of action. Hospital leadership is in a much better position to evaluate growth strategies after a lean transformation because they have experienced what lean principles can do for an organization. Mapping the value stream for each product and service family identifies where future opportunities exist.

IMPETUS TO ENGAGE

Although a lean transformation is a massive undertaking, the need for such a transformation has never more apparent. It's not for the faint of heart. Before you decide that a lean transformation requires too much effort, consider the words of Thomas Edison:

- *"Many of life's failures are experienced by people who did not realize how close they were to success when they gave up."* After reading this book you may be excited and ready to engage your organization in a lean transformation, but things will come up. Reports are due, problems must be solved, budgets must be established, demands are made on your time, you get caught up in something else, and the initiative is placed on a back burner, possibly forever. Subconsciously, you have given up before you even began. Your proximity to success has never been greater than it is right now, as you are reading these words. You must not let yourself be sidetracked. You are a decision away from an exciting, promising, and rewarding opportunity right now. Don't let it slip away!

- *"The three things that are most essential to achievement are common sense, hard work, and stick-to-it-iv-ness."* The tools and principles described in this book are based on common sense. It is well known that common sense is an uncommon phenomenon. The application of these concepts is difficult; it requires hard work and tenacity. A lean transformation combines the three elements Mr. Edison specified in this quote as being most essential to achievement.

- *"If we all did the things we are really capable of doing, we would literally astound ourselves."* We would not only astound ourselves but also those around us. Any organization is capable of becoming a lean organization—regardless of size, regardless of funds, regardless of location, regardless of anything else. This is an opportunity unlike any other. Take on the challenge, roll up your sleeves, and make the commitment to become a lean organization.

Astound yourself!

GLOSSARY

affinity diagram—A planning tool used to organize ideas by placing each idea on a separate card and grouping them in creative ways.

andon—Andon is the Japanese word for "light." An andon is most commonly a light or an audible signal, but it may be any signal used to bring attention to a particular situation.

batch-and-queue—A production method that entails making large quantities of parts that are passed along to the next downstream process, only to sit in queue.

business-value-added—Process steps that do not contribute directly to providing the product or service that the patient/customer desires, but which are required or necessary for the product/services to be provided.

cause-and-effect diagram—A statistical tool used to demonstrate the relationship between possible causes and a particular effect.

chuku-chuku—Chuku is the Japanese word for "load." Chuku-Chuku means load-load, which describes a process that requires only loading and no effort for unloading.

combination sheet—The combination sheet combines manual, walking, automatic, and waiting times in a graphical, easy-to-read representation of the process.

continuous improvement—The never-ending cycle of improvement that involves everyone in the organization.

Cp—A numerical value that defines the ability of the process to produce data that falls within the range created by the upper and lower specification limits.

Cpk—A numerical value that identifies whether the process is centered within the specification limits and thereby acceptable.

cycle time—The amount of time necessary to complete one cycle of an operation or a process.

decision matrix—See *prioritization matrix*.

Deming cycle—See *Plan, Do, Check, Act*.

design of experiment (DOE)—A tool that allows a team to determine the effect of different proposed problem solutions on the process output.

DMAIC—The methodology used in Six Sigma implementation. DMAIC denotes the five phases of implementation: define, measure, analyze, improve, and control.

DOE—See *design of experiment*.

downstream process—A process that is subsequent to another process in the value stream.

DPMO—Defects per million opportunities.

failure mode and effects analysis (FMEA)—A systematic method for recognizing, evaluating, documenting, and prioritizing the magnitude of potential failure modes and the source of the potential failures.

fishbone diagram—See *cause-and-effect diagram*.

Five S (5S)—A lean tool targeted at perpetuating a neat, clean, and organized workplace. The five Ss are Sort, Straighten, Scrub, Standardize, and Sustain.

Five Whys—A method for determining the root cause of a problem by asking "why?" at least five times.

flow—Progressive, continuous process steps along the value stream. Flow is accomplished through the elimination of constraints or obstacles that impede the movement of patient or product from one operation or process to the next.

gemba—A Japanese word that means "the scene of the action," more loosely interpreted as the location where the process is performed.

heijunka—See *level loading*.

histogram—A graphical representation of the frequency distribution of a data set.

Ishikawa diagram—See *cause-and-effect diagram*.

jidoka—Jidoka is automation with a human touch. Most commonly a machine with a device for detecting defects and a mechanism to stop the machine should a defect occur.

Just-In-Time (JIT)—A methodology for supplying a process with what is needed, when it is needed, in the quantity needed. JIT eliminates the need for inventory between process steps.

kaikaku—The Japanese word for "radical improvement," the opposite of kaizen, which is continuous incremental improvement

kaizen—A Japanese word meaning "change for the better" or continuous incremental improvement.

kanban—The Japanese word for "signboard." A kanban is a device used to signal the need for replenishment.

lead time—The time it takes to process one patient/product through the entire value stream from beginning to end.

lean—A methodology spawned by the Toyota Production System (TPS) aimed at the elimination of non-value-added operations in the workplace in order to create flow and quick response to customer demand.

lean event—The dedication of a team of individuals whose sole purpose is to implement lean tools and concepts in a targeted area. A typical lean event lasts three to five days.

level loading—A method of sequencing product or service orders in a cyclical arrangement in order to provide an even distribution of that product or service.

mean—The average value of a set of numbers. Calculated by summing the numbers in the set and then dividing the sum by the total of numbers in the set.

measurement system analysis (MSA)—An analysis method that verifies the validity of the measurement device as well as the repeatability and reproducibility engendered by the person or people obtaining the data set.

mistake proofing—See *poka-yoke*.

MSA—See measurement system analysis.

muda—The Japanese word for waste, often used to describe non-value-added process steps.

non-value-added—A description of process steps that do not contribute directly to providing the product or service the patient/customer desires; not required or necessary.

objective—The goal, the desired end result of a given plan.

one-piece flow—Providing one complete service or product at a time through the value stream without interruption; the opposite of a batch-and-queue method.

operation— A particular task performed in order to provide a service or produce a product.

PDCA—See *Plan, Do, Check, Act.*

percent load chart—A tool for determining whether the workload is well balanced and identifying staffing levels needed to meet takt time.

Plan, Do, Check, Act (PDCA)—A cycle which, when applied to a process, allows managers to identify and change the parts of the process that need improvements. A cycle of steps designed to drive continuous improvement.

poka-yoke—Mistake proofing; derived from two Japanese words: yokeru, which means to avoid, and poka, which means errors.

prioritization matrix—A tool used for prioritizing tasks based on weighted criteria.

process—A string of discrete operations required to provide a service or produce a product.

process capability—See *Cp and Cpk.*

process map—A map showing the sequence of events categorized as Service, Preparation, Transportation, or Queue.

process sequence—The sequence in which activities are performed by one or more people to complete one process cycle time.

pull—A system in which a patient or product advances from an upstream process step only when a need is signaled from the downstream process step. The customer is then said to be pulling value from the supplier.

quick changeover—A set-up time-reduction methodology. See *single minute exchange of die.*

root cause—The critical underlying cause of a problem or a failure.

root-cause analysis—Any of several different methods employed to learn why a particular failure or problem exists (See Five Whys, cause-and-effect diagram, and failure mode and effects analysis).

sensei—The Japanese word for teacher, the term is often used in regard to a consultant or an in-house expert in lean principles.

Seven Wastes—Seven areas identified by Taichii Ohno where non-value-added operations are prevalent. They are Delay, Over Processing, Inventory, Transportation, Motion, Over Producing, and Making Defects.

single minute exchange of die (SMED)—A quick-changeover methodology to reduce equipment downtime and optimize efficiency.

Six Sigma—A data-driven approach to quality improvement that employs statistical analysis to reduce or eliminate process variation and focus attention on customer needs.

SMED—See *single minute exchange of die*.

spaghetti chart—A term used to describe a standard worksheet.

standard deviation—The square root of the average squared distance of each value of a set of numbers from the mean.

standard work—The most effective combination of activities that will minimize non-value-added activities while providing high quality care.

standard work in process (SWIP)—The minimum number of patients or products required to ensure flow by maintaining the process sequence.

standard worksheet—A form used to document the existing work sequence by tracing, on the form, the path of the person or people performing the process tasks.

standardize—To update methods and procedures in order to ensure that everyone knows what is expected.

strategic deployment session—A session in which a team of individuals work together to establish specific goals relative to the strategic plan.

SWIP—See *standard work in process*.

SWOT—An acronym for Strengths, Weaknesses, Opportunities, and Threats.

takt time—The rate of patient/customer demand.

time observation sheet—A form employed to break down a process into individual operations and observe how much time is required to complete each step.

total employee involvement—A discipline that encourages total participation of people at the operating level.

Toyota Production System—See *lean*.

TPS—See *Toyota Production System*.

upstream process—A process that precedes another process in the value stream.

value added—An operation or process step that contributes directly to providing the product or service the patient/customer desires.

value stream—All the action that takes place to bring a product or service through to completion.

visual control—A device used to share information without speaking.

work cell—A grouping of people and equipment dedicated to a common operation or test.

work sequence—The sequence in which activities are performed by one person to complete one cycle time.

BIBLIOGRAPHY

Beals, G. (1996). *Thomas Edison "Quotes."* Retrieved December 20, 2005, from http://www.thomasedison.com/edquote.htm

Blue Cross and Blue Shield Association. (2004). *What are the major factors of rising healthcare costs?* Retrieved December 21, 2005, from http://www.fepblue.org/faq/faqhealthcarecosts.html#1

Brown, C. (Writer) (1940). Edison the man. In John W. Considine, Jr. (Producer). USA.

Chase, R. B. & Aquilano, N. J. (1995). *Production and operations management.* Chicago, IL: Richard D. Irwin, Inc.

Committee on Quality of Healthcare in America, Institute of Medicine. (2000). *To err is human: building a safer medical system.* Washington, D. C.: National Academy Press.

Council on Graduate Medical Education. (2005). *Physician workforce policy guidelines for the United States, 2000-2020.* Retrieved December 20, 2005, from http://www.cogme.gov/report16.htm#sop

Deming, W. E. (1986). *Out of crisis.* Cambridge, MA: MIT Center for Advanced Engineering Study.

Fisher, D. (2000, December 11, 2000). The man who would save health care. *Forbes,* pp.180-188.

Goldratt, E. M. & Cox, J. (1992). *The goal.* Great Barrington, MA: North River Press, Inc.

Gonick, L. & Smith, W. (1993). *The cartoon guide to statistics.* New York, NY: HarperCollins Publishers, Inc.

Healthcare Financial Management Association (HFMA). (2005). *Updating charity care policies and processes can help you meet the rising tide of uninsured patients.* Retrieved December 20, 2005, from http://www.hfma.org/publications/know_newsletter/101905.htm

Health Resources and Services Administration. (2002). *Projected supply, demand, and shortages of registered nurses: 2000-2020.* Retrieved December 20, 2005, from http://bhpr.hrsa.gov/healthworkforce/reports/behindrnprojections/behind shortage.htm

Henderson, B. A. & Larco, J. L. (1999). Lean transformation: *How to change your business into a lean enterprise.* Richmond, VA: The Oaklea Press.

Hiroyuki, H. (1989). *JIT Implementation Manual: The complete guide to just-in-time manufacturing.* Tokyo, Japan: JIT Management Laboratory Company, Ltd.

Hiroyuki, H. (1995). *5 Pillars of the visual workplace.* Portland, OR: Productivity Press.

Joint Commission on Accreditation of Healthcare Organization. (2005). *Overview of 2007 hospital leadership chapter (Revisions in Progress).* Retrieved December 28, 2005, from http://www.jointcommission.org/NR/rdonlyres/F42AF828-7248-48C0-B4E6-BA18E719A87C/0/06_hap_accred_stds.pdf

Kotter, J. P. (1996). *Leading change.* Boston, MA: Harvard Business School Press.

Martin D. Merry, M. D. (2003). Healthcare's need for revolutionary change. *ASQ, 36*(9), 31-35.

National Coalition on Health Care. (2004). *Health insurance cost.* Retrieved December 21, 2005, from http://www.nchc.org/facts/cost.shtml

Plsek, P. E. & Onnias, A. (1989). *Quality improvement tools* (Vol. 4). Wilton, CT: Juran Institute, Inc.

Rother, M. & Shook, John. (1998). *Learning to see: Value stream mapping to add value and eliminate muda* (Vol. 1.0). Brookline, MA: The Lean Enterprise Institute.

Shingo, S. (1983). *A revolution in manufacturing: The SMED system.* Portland, OR: Productivity Press.

Shingo, S. (1986). *Zero quality control: Source inspection and the poka-yoke system.* Portland, OR: Productivity Press.

Toyota Motor Company Sales Company, Ltd. (1995-2005). *The history of Toyota.* Retrieved December 20, 2005, from http://www.toyota.co.jp/en/history/1950.html

U. S. News & World Report (July 18, 2005). *America's Best Hospitals*, pp. 112-140

Wikipedia, the free encyclopedia. (2005). *World War II*. Retrieved December 20, 2005, from http://en.wikipedia.org/wiki/World_War_II

Williams, B. R. (1996). *Manufacturing for survival: The how-to guide for practitioners and managers*. Reading, MA: Addison-Wesley Publishing Company.

Womack, J. P., Jones, D. T., & Roos, D. (1990). *The machine that changed the world*. New York, NY: HarperCollins Publishers

Womack, J. P, & Jones, D. T. (1996). *Lean thinking: Banish waste and create wealth in your corporation*. New York, NY: Simon & Schuster.

Yale New Haven Hospital. (2005). *About Yale-New Haven Hospital*. Retrieved January, 10, 2006, from http://www.ynhh.org/general/general.html

APPENDIX

Outpatient Blood Draw Example for Value Stream Mapping

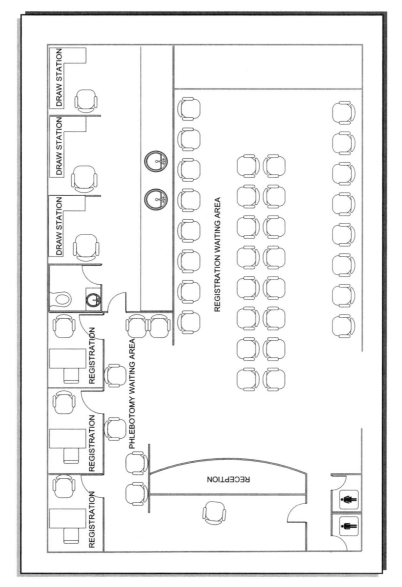

The laboratory outpatient blood draw department of University Hospital has three registration offices and three blood draw stations, as shown in the floor plan above. The process is staffed by a volunteer receptionist, two registrars, and one phlebotomist; it is open from 6:30 a.m. to 3:00 p.m. The staff gets two fifteen-minute breaks and takes a half hour lunch. Patients are seen on a first-come, first-served basis. Although the department opens at 6:30 a.m., fasting patients begin to arrive at 6:00 a.m. so they can get in and out quickly. On any given day, the number of patients waiting for the department to open ranges from zero to twelve, the number of patients waiting for registration ranges from zero to twenty, and the number of patients waiting for phlebotomy ranges from zero to six. On average, patients wait 90 seconds for reception, 12 minutes for registration, and 6 minutes for phlebotomy. The department processes 100 patients a day, and the process cycle times are as follows:

Reception	1 minute, 30 seconds (90 seconds)
Registration	4 minutes (240 seconds)
Phlebotomy	3 minutes (180 seconds)

Prior to the patient's arrival, the doctor's office faxes test requests to the Laboratory Services department; this information is entered into the database manually by a Laboratory clerk. The registrar obtains the orders from the database during registration. Upon completion of registration, the data is uploaded to the database and specimen labels print out in the phlebotomy area.

At the end of each day the specimens are transported to the lab for testing and the results are faxed to the doctor's offices.

This department has been targeted for improvement because of the rise in patient complaints related to waiting. Some patients have waited more than an hour to be registered and have their blood drawn. Doctor's offices have been complaining about the poor turnaround time from order to results. The Laboratory director has put in a request for an additional phlebotomist to eliminate the waiting problem.

INDEX

NOTES